Sudden Unexpected Death in Epilepsy

continuing the global conversation

Edited by
Denise Chapman
Rosemary Panelli
Jane Hanna
Tamzin Jeffs

Epilepsy Australia Ltd
Epilepsy Bereaved
SUDEP Aware

First published in 2011 by:

Epilepsy Australia Ltd
818 Burke Road
Camberwell Victoria 3124
Australia
www.epilepsyaustralia.net
email: sudep@epilepsyaustralia.net

Epilepsy Bereaved
PO Box 112
Wantage
Oxon OX12 8XT
United Kingdom
www.sudep.org
email: contact@epilepsybereaved.org.uk

SUDEP Aware
Suite 350
283 Danforth Avenue
Toronto, Ontario M4K 1N2
Canada
www.sudepaware.org
email: info@sudepaware.org

ISBN 978-0-9758011-1-6

This publication is funded in part by Epilepsy Australia's SUDEP Research & Education Fund.

Printed for free distribution.

Cover Image by Jenny Solomon, Dreamstimes.com

Referencing

Sudden Unexpected Death in Epilepsy: continuing the global conversation should be cited as
follows:

Chapman, D, Panelli, R, Hanna, J & Jeffs, T, eds. 2011, Sudden unexpected death in epilepsy:
continuing the global conversation, Epilepsy Australia, Epilepsy Bereaved & SUDEP Aware,
Camberwell, Australia.

Contents

Contents

Contents

Foreword by Mike Glynn

SUDEP was largely 'forgotten' by both the medical and the voluntary sectors until the late 1990s. Such deaths were not understood, and they were largely accepted as an inevitable part of a difficult condition. Those working in the field of epilepsy were not inclined to dwell on this negative outcome for fear of promoting anxiety in those who live with the condition, and their families. When organizations like Epilepsy Bereaved UK began to ask questions about SUDEP, their persistence brought the issue out of the shadows. Research projects sprang up, an understanding of SUDEP began to grow, and with it insights into possible risk factors.

Current evidence indicates that most doctors working with epilepsy are now knowledgeable about SUDEP, yet many are not warning their patients about the risks. While all patients have individual needs requiring careful judgment when imparting information, the goal should be to work with each patient, drawing on the available information to protect them from any potential risks that can be identified from the outset.

The biggest obstacle blocking progress in the provision of SUDEP information appears to be the 'right not to know' argument being put forward as a reason for not informing patients. It may take litigation or legislation to remove this but it would be far preferable if an internal guideline could be produced within the epilepsy medical world to deal with this issue.

Since *Sudden Unexpected Death in Epilepsy: a global conversation* appeared in 2005, there has been good news on SUDEP, including a joint task force report by the American Epilepsy Society and Epilepsy Foundation, and reports to the UK parliament by the Joint Epilepsy Council and the Australian parliament by the Joint Epilepsy Council of Australia. Last year, the first Clinical Lead for Epilepsy in Ireland made the reduction of SUDEP and other epilepsy deaths his number one priority. In addition, SUDEP is now a growth area in epilepsy research. However much remains to be done on prevention and risk communication. This new edition of the 'global conversation' is a welcome resource to assist in the challenge to reduce epilepsy deaths.

I congratulate the editors and all of the authors on this latest production.

Mike Glynn
President
International Bureau for Epilepsy

Foreword by Solomon L. Moshé

Epilepsy is a very common disease affecting 50 million people worldwide. It is more common than multiple sclerosis, cerebral palsy, muscular dystrophy and Parkinson disease combined. Epilepsy represents more than recurrence of seizures because it is associated with significant comorbidities. Most importantly, over the last few years studies have demonstrated that people with epilepsy have a shorter lifespan with two to three fold increase in mortality, including a 24 fold increase in SUDEP. It has been reported that one in 100 people with epilepsy per year may suffer SUDEP, especially those suffering from frequent convulsive seizures. During the past year several papers have been published further documenting the circumstances under which SUDEP occurs, but this volume provides a unique opportunity to summarize state of the art information, as well as to incorporate testimonials from people whose relatives have suddenly died from epilepsy.

To date, the ILAE and IBE are promoting key synergistic partnerships with national and international governments, NGOs, foundations and other professional organizations assisting patients with epilepsy, as well as consumer groups to develop strategies towards dissemination of vital information related to the decreased life expectancy of people with epilepsy, and particularly, SUDEP. It is very clear that there is an urgent need to collect more information, and this volume serves this purpose by reaching out to all and by providing the latest findings.

However, we also need to explore ways to prevent SUDEP, and this can only be achieved through effective translational research identifying the contributing factors of this devastating condition, and to find cures. By working as a team we should be able to achieve our goal whereby epilepsy and its comorbidities are a thing of the past.

This volume, six years after the first edition of *Sudden Unexpected Death in Epilepsy: a global conversation* was introduced, brings the field forward by leaps and bounds. Both the editors and authors should be congratulated for this very informative and valuable publication.

Solomon L. Moshé, MD
President
International League Against Epilepsy

Acknowledgements

The publication of *Sudden Unexpected Death in Epilepsy: a global conversation*, in 2005, prompted gratifying international endorsement. By presenting a succinct picture of SUDEP, and combining science with the human experience in an accessible style, the book proved to be a resource of value to both health professionals and the general community.

Six years later, although causes remain elusive, evidence supports SUDEP risk reduction strategies. Health policy changes reflect some growth in the understanding of epilepsy-related death, and there has also been a small increase in community awareness. However, deaths still occur in families with no knowledge that such a tragedy can occur bringing not only grief but also endless regret that knowledge might have prevented the death.

Many SUDEP questions have not yet been answered and global debate continues. The need for clear and concise information on this topic is ongoing, prompting us to 'continue the conversation' with a second book. The editorial partnership has been strengthened with SUDEP Aware (Canada) joining Epilepsy Australia and Epilepsy Bereaved (UK), and by the International Bureau for Epilepsy endorsing and supporting the publication as part of its golden jubilee celebrations.

We thank all our authors for their encouragement and their generous contribution to this project. They have given of their time and expertise freely. The growth in SUDEP research has been pleasing but in this small publication it is very difficult to offer a complete overview of developments. We apologise for any omissions and we have included an extensive bibliography to assist readers who wish to explore the topic in more depth.

Sixteen bereaved families have honoured us with contributions. Their stories offer insights into lives lived with epilepsy, the search for quality care, and the challenges of balancing the risks of epilepsy against quality of life. Their stories are a tribute to their loved ones and we thank them for their faith in this book.

Thank you to everyone who has made this project possible. Our commitment to the global conversation will not end with this publication. We plan to continue the discussion and debate and invite you to follow us at www.sudepglobalconversation.com

Denise Chapman, Rosemary Panelli, Jane Hanna and Tamzin Jeffs

Part 1.

facing the facts

Epilepsy kills

Epilepsy is often seen as a benign condition in which people have seizures but not much more; nothing could be further from the truth. Epilepsy is indeed a malignant condition which carries a high risk of premature death in those people who carry on having seizures – who are without full control. Almost all studies have shown this, and the increase in the risk of early death is an important component of the burden of epilepsy.

So what brings this about? What are the determinants of this increased risk of premature mortality? In the initial years after diagnosis, it seems that the same problem that causes the epilepsy (such as cerebrovascular disease or brain tumour) is also responsible for the increased risk of death. Amongst people with chronic epilepsy, however, epilepsy itself is the major culprit, as people with the condition may die as a result of an accident (such as drowning) brought on by a seizure, or from status epilepticus, but particularly from Sudden Unexpected Death in Epilepsy (SUDEP).

What is SUDEP? The definition of SUDEP is well known and accepted as an unexpected death in a person with epilepsy in whom no clear causes for death are found despite full post mortem examination. It is a baffling condition which brings sorrow and bereavement to many families every year. Indeed, in the UK, it is likely that over 1,000 people with epilepsy die suddenly and unexpectedly every year and this is more than die from AIDS, for instance, or asthma. Little is known about the precise causes of SUDEP although it is now accepted that it is likely to be triggered by a seizure as, almost invariably, it seems to happen in the aftermath of a seizure.

A number of possible mechanisms for SUDEP have been suggested and currently there are many on-going research projects trying to elucidate the underlying causes. Potential causes that have been discussed and are being investigated include cardiac mechanisms, respiratory failure, and autonomic failure. We may well eventually find that there is no single mechanism but rather a combination of several mechanisms which may act and interact in different ways in different people. Knowing the mechanisms for SUDEP will help to clarify the search for effective preventative measures to stop its occurrence, thus decreasing the burden of epilepsy.

Josemir W. Sander
Professor of Neurology & Clinical Epilepsy
UCL Institute of Neurology, London, UK.
Epilepsy Institute in the Netherlands Foundation, Netherlands.

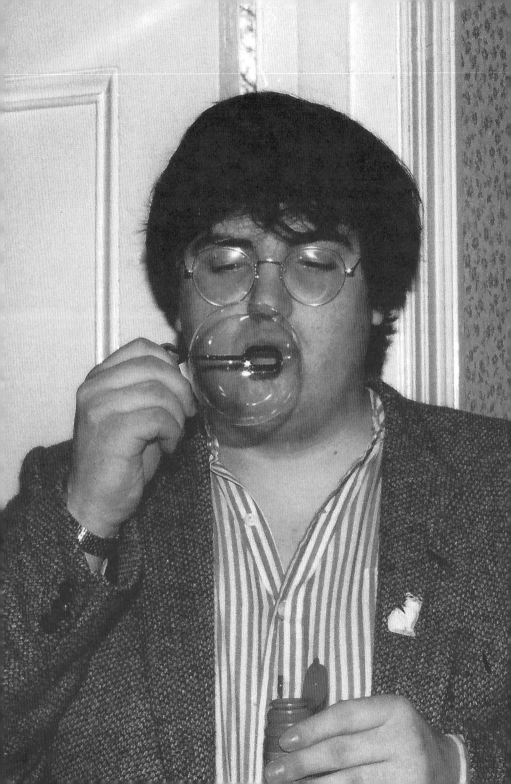

William

People do not die from epilepsy. That is what we were told when William died as a result of a seizure in 1988. William had his first seizure at 17½ and his last at 22 years. In between he gained four A Levels, a place at Oxford, a degree in English and planned to become a teacher.

The money that friends and relations donated was given to what was then the British Epilepsy Association, now Epilepsy Action, to be used to fund a booklet. Over the next few years we collected more money and produced Epilepsy and the Young Adult, which is still in print today.

In 1994 The Guardian Newspaper published an article about a boy called Matthew. It took courage to read it. That was the first time I realized that there were other deaths like William's but as a result of this article I met Matthew's mother Catherine Brookes, Jane Hanna, who had lost her partner Alan, his mother, and Sue Kelk, whose daughter Natalie had also died. Together we founded, in 1996, the charity Epilepsy Bereaved. By then we had already been in touch with another sixty families.

The aims of the charity then and now, are to console and inform families where there has been a death and to give bereaved families the opportunity to meet. The charity began to raise awareness in the UK and around the world. It also encourages and funds research into sudden death from epilepsy.

Our first major achievement, with the help of doctors Stephen Brown and Lina Nashef, was to convene the first ever international workshop on Sudden Death from Epilepsy. The thirty speakers and seventy discussants came from all over the world. It was during this meeting that Sudden Unexpected Death from Epilepsy (SUDEP) was defined.

Our second major success was to get funding for the first National Sentinel Audit into Epilepsy Deaths. Published in 2002, it proved that there were nearly a thousand UK deaths a year as a result of epilepsy, of which 500 were SUDEPs. It also showed that possibly 42% of these were preventable. Figures now show that there are, on average, three deaths from epilepsy every day in the UK.

We had, and still have, a hard job persuading epilepsy organizations and even some professionals to talk about the risk, however small, of Sudden Death, yet in fifteen years we have grown from a small organization with one part-time member of staff, to one with worldwide connections, caring for nearly a thousand families.

So now we know that people can die as result of a seizure. I wish I had known that when William died, as it would have been a comfort to talk to other families who had suffered in the same way.

Jennifer Preston

SUDEP: definitions and classification

SUDEP is a category of deaths in people with epilepsy and not a condition. It is likely that this category includes cases with different mechanisms and circumstances. Definitions for what is included in this category are needed as they allow for comparisons between different studies and monitoring trends. Two SUDEP definitions/classification systems (Nashef 1997, Annegers 1997) have been in use for more than 10 years. The Nashef definition below, focuses on strictly defined cases with negative post mortem, while the Annegers definition additionally gives guidance on classifying the many cases where information is incomplete, with definite, probable and possible categories. Both are useful. The strictly defined category may be particularly helpful in studying mechanisms while broader categories need to be taken into account in epidemiological work, especially in population based work, where information is often lacking. These complementary definitions together have provided the basis for classification of SUDEP cases in most studies. The time has come to revisit these with the aim of proposing one definition/classification system (Nashef et al. in preparation). Ideally, this would extend, clarify and unify those in use while maintaining consistency with most published research in the last two decades.

SUDEP: Sudden, unexpected, witnessed or unwitnessed, non traumatic and non drowning death in an individual with epilepsy, with or without evidence for a seizure and excluding documented status epilepticus, where post mortem examination does not reveal a toxicologic or anatomic cause for death (Nashef 1997).

While the description above, with some minor qualification, would still apply to definite SUDEP, with the probable category unchanged (fulfils all criteria for definite SUDEP but without a post mortem examination), the possible category requires review. Currently, it includes both cases where there is a competing cause for death with those where there is insufficient information to classify the death (Annegers 1997). As a consequence of this ambiguity, the possible category has not been useful in epidemiological studies and often only the definite and probable SUDEP categories are used to calculate incidence. There are also situations where death may be due to the combined or synergistic effect of both the epilepsy and a concomitant condition and these too need to be considered.

Other issues that need to be addressed include:

■ *The acronym SUDEP and what is stands for.* 'Unexpected' is favoured over 'Unexplained'. The latter has given rise to some confusion as, while it can be taken to mean a negative post mortem and no structural cause for death, some have wrongly understood it to mean no evidence of a terminal seizure. Furthermore, as a better understanding of non-structural mechanisms emerges, its use becomes less appropriate.

■ *More clarity in relation to including within the category of SUDEP the vast majority of cases where body position may have contributed to air not getting in freely and not as a separate category of 'asphyxia' or 'suffocation'.* Although respiratory obstruction is likely to be a contributory remedial factor in some cases of SUDEP, this happens within the context of coma caused by the seizure. This results in lack of corrective action to remedy any obstruction. In addition, many patients stop breathing during a seizure due to central mechanisms (central apnea). In any individual case, the relative contribution of central apnea, which very frequently occurs in seizures, and positional airway obstruction is difficult to establish and separating cases into one or other is generally not workable.

■ *The clarification of the time from any witnessed terminal event to death.* Some SUDEP deaths may not be immediate after a terminal collapse or seizure. As most cases are unwitnessed, any time specified, which would need to be relatively short, is by necessity arbitrary.

■ *The definition of near SUDEP where a resuscitation procedure is deemed to have prevented death following cardio-respiratory arrest.* For such an event to be classified as near-SUDEP, it needs to satisfy the other criteria required for SUDEP, that is without a structural or toxicological cause for the collapse found on investigation of the collapse.

Classification systems are by their nature to some extent arbitrary, particularly in a situation where most deaths are unwitnessed and where there is no pathological diagnosis of SUDEP. Nevertheless, the older definitions have been workable and stood the test of time, and any unified proposal will need to fit in with the older classifications and be easily applicable and useful in different studies and for monitoring purposes.

Lina Nashef
King's College Hospital, London, UK.

SUDEP: incidence and predisposing factors

Sudden unexpected death is a well established concept in cardiology, describing a situation where a person in a reasonable state of health and under benign circumstances suddenly dies, usually due to a cardiac condition such as a fatal arrhythmia. Although rare, sudden death can hit anyone in the population.

For people with epilepsy the average risk of dying suddenly and unexpectedly has been estimated to more than 20 times greater than in the general population based on a study from the US. This fact is the background to the more specific term Sudden Unexpected Death in Epilepsy (SUDEP), referring to sudden death in a person with epilepsy. A recent 40 years follow-up of children once diagnosed with epilepsy suggests that SUDEP may account for approximately 30% of all deaths in people with epilepsy (Sillanpää & Shinnar 2010).

However, the risk of SUDEP varies markedly, almost 100-fold, between epilepsy patients. The lowest risk is seen among people with newly diagnosed epilepsy where SUDEP is truly rare. Studies have estimated the risk to be in the order of 1 in 10,000 person years, i.e. one can expect on average one case of SUDEP if 1,000 persons were followed during 10 years after their seizure onset. Greatest risks are found among those with severe chronic epilepsy. As an example, the SUDEP risk has been estimated to 5-10 in 1,000 person years for patients with refractory epilepsy and who are candidates for epilepsy surgery.

SUDEP has been recognized at least since the 19th century but we do not know if the rates have changed with time. Nor do we know if there are any regional differences in the incidence. Researchers in the UK have investigated if there is a seasonal variation in the risk and found no evidence for that.

Several studies have tried to find factors predisposing to SUDEP (risk factors) in order to identify people with particularly high risks. This is usually done in so called case-control studies that compare different characteristics of cases that have died in SUDEP with those of people with epilepsy who have not suffered SUDEP.

A Task Force of the International League Against Epilepsy (ILAE) recently pooled data from four major such case-control studies from the UK, Sweden and US (Hesdorffer et al. 2011). Altogether 289 SUDEP cases and 958 living epilepsy controls were included in this combined analysis. The risk of SUDEP was found to be 1.4-fold higher in males compared to females, 1.7 fold higher in those with onset of their epilepsy at young age (before 16 years) compared to those with onset between 16 and 60 years, and two fold higher among those with a duration of epilepsy of more than 15 years. The most important risk factor was frequency of generalized tonic-clonic seizures. Compared to people without tonic-clonic seizures, 1-2 such seizures/year was associated with a 3-fold increase in risk, 3-50 seizures/year with an 8-9- fold increase. The risk was almost 15-fold higher for those with > 50 tonic-clonic seizures/year. Other studies have indicated that the SUDEP risk may be 20 times higher among people with epilepsy who continue to have seizures compared with those who are seizure-free.

The role of treatment with antiepileptic drugs has also been assessed. Lack of treatment has been associated with increased risk in a study from UK. Combination therapy (polytherapy) with antiepileptic drugs had a 3-fold higher risk compared with those on monotherapy in the combined ILAE analysis. It is, however, unclear if the greater risk with polytherapy merely reflects risks with a more severe epilepsy, or if it is due to the drug treatment as such. There is no conclusive evidence of greater risks associated with the use of individual specific antiepileptic drugs.

Torbjörn Tomson
Professor of Neurology
Karolinska University Hospital, Stockholm, Sweden.

SUDEP and childhood-onset epilepsy

SUDEP is a common but often unrecognized diagnosis mostly ascribed to an epileptic seizure. SUDEP is defined by Annegers (1997) as having a sudden death with no evidence of a seizure, no other cause of death, and confirmation by autopsy for definite SUDEP. There is another definition of Nashef (1997) which also includes probable or definite seizures though excludes definite status epilepticus. There are few studies about SUDEP from cohorts of people with epilepsy followed for tens of years, from childhood through adulthood.

Our study subjects with epilepsy (N=245) were a representative cohort of an unselected general child population followed up regularly for almost 40 years for mortality including SUDEP (Sillanpää & Shinnar 2010). We applied the definition of Annegers (1997) for SUDEP as the primary analysis but also looked at it using the definition of Nashef (1997).

During the follow-up period, 60 patients died yielding an overall case fatality of 24.5% and mortality rate of 6.90/1000 patient-years. SUDEP was the cause of death in 18/60(30%) according to the criteria of Annegers, but in 23/60(38%), when probable or definite seizures, but not status epilepticus, were included in agreements with the definition of Nashef (1997). More than half (55%) were epilepsy-related deaths, and of them, SUDEP was the most common cause (in 30%) followed by definite or probable seizure (15%) and accidental drowning (10%). Of 18 cases of SUDEP, 15(83%) were autopsied and are, therefore, definite SUDEP. Of these, 7 patients had an idiopathic or cryptogenic epilepsy and the remaining 11 a symptomatic epilepsy. The median age at death was 25.7 years (range 4-49 years) for all cases, and 17.9 years (range 4-49 years) with symptomatic epilepsy. Only 2 of 18 patients with SUDEP died in childhood (at age 4 and 6 years, respectively), and both of them had a symptomatic epilepsy.

Over the 40-year follow-up period, the risk of SUDEP (Annegers 1997) was 7% (95%CI 5%-12%) overall, and the annual risk was 0.18%. The risk was 12% (95%CI 8%-20%) for those patients who were not in five-year terminal remission off medications. The risk for SUDEP in patients with idiopathic/cryptogenic epilepsy was 5% (95%CI 2%-11%) for all cases and 15% (95%CI 7%-31%) for cases who were not in five-year terminal remission without medications. Thus, patients who fail to achieve terminal remission are at substantially higher risk for SUDEP than those with terminal remission. On multivariable analysis, the absence of 5-year terminal remission was the only significant predictor of SUDEP. The hazard ratio was 5.0-fold (95%CI 1.2-20.1). Patients with drug-resistant epilepsy who have become seizure-free after surgery have a lower risk for SUDEP than those with no remission (Sperling et al. 1999) and, on the other hand, patients on the waiting list for epilepsy surgery have a very high risk of death from SUDEP (Tomson, Nashef & Ryvlin et al. 2008).

Considering the high autopsy rate (83%), we could probably ascertain all the cases of SUDEP. While an overall childhood mortality in epilepsy is higher than in adulthood (Zielinski 1974, Hauser, Annegers & Elvback 1980) the mortality does not occur in childhood. Other studies of childhood onset epilepsy reported low rates of SUDEP and, essentially, the deaths occurred only in children with symptomatic epilepsy (Berg et al. 2004, Camfield & Camfield 2005, Shinnar, O'Dell & Berg 2005). The results of our study are consistent with those studies. However, they did not follow the children into adulthood which is when the high rates of SUDEP occur. The peak incidence for SUDEP is reported to be 20–40 years (Ficker et al. 1998), which was the case in our data.

In conclusion, in those with childhood onset epilepsy, the risk for SUDEP is low in childhood but dramatically rises in adult life. The risk is particularly high in adults with epilepsy who are not in five-year terminal remission. While not a randomized trial, the results clearly argue that attaining complete control of seizures is an important goal. While, those with self limited childhood epilepsy syndromes such as benign Rolandic epilepsy and childhood absence do not appear to be at significant risk for SUDEP, we must be cognizant that childhood onset epilepsy syndromes that persist into adulthood are associated with a significant risk of SUDEP in addition to the other comorbidities that may be present (Sillanpää et al. 1998). When children with epilepsy reach adolescence and are not attaining remission, a discussion of SUDEP should take place when appropriate. The risk of SUDEP is one of the factors that argues for aggressive management of epilepsy to attain complete control including use of newer agents and surgery when appropriate.

Matti Sillanpää
Departments of Pediatrics, Neurology and Public Health
University of Turku, Finland.

Shlomo Shinnar
Professor of Neurology & Pediatrics
Albert Einstein College of Medicine, Bronx, NY, USA.

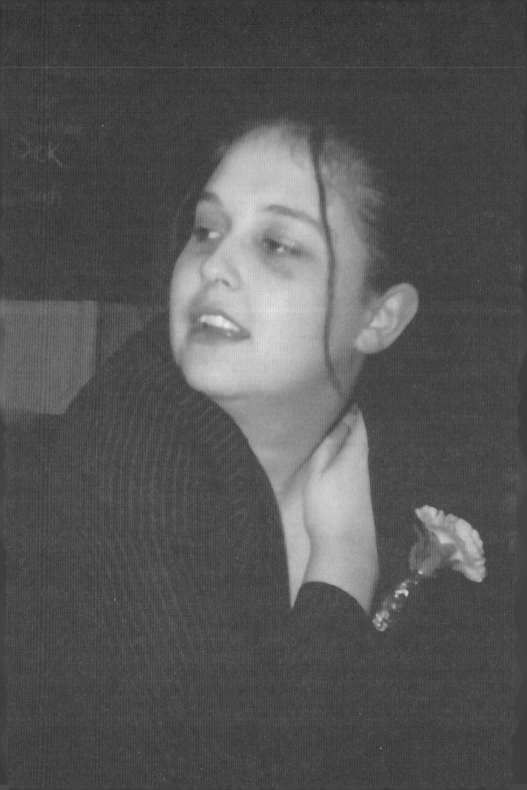

Karen

Karen was 10 when she suffered her first epileptic seizure and it was shortly after that she was diagnosed with generalized epilepsy.

On 7 September 2008, I received a call that no parent could imagine or should receive; my 26 year old daughter had been found dead in her apartment.

The cause of death was SUDEP; something I had never heard of. Like most parents in my position I wondered if I had done enough. What could I have done differently?

Although Karen had up to 15 seizures a day, she was a very independent young lady, who never asked for any support and she lived her life to the full despite her condition.

On clearing out her apartment I found a diary with a wish list where Karen had written that she wanted a seizure alert dog. Although this may not have saved her life, it would have made an amazing difference to her life. My guilt was immense, but not understanding what had happened was the worst thing. I never imagined that she could die so suddenly; I had no idea of the risks associated with epilepsy.

I found it hard to admit that I needed some support – someone who may help me to understand and answer some of the questions that were eating away at me. Talking to Epilepsy Bereaved helped me and I began to realize that maybe I could channel my grief into something positive; it was too late for Karen but maybe I could do something that would change things for others.

It was then that I began to write the play 'Karen's Wishes'. Our story is so much like many others and I wanted to share it with as many people as possible. I knew it was a massive task but, with the help of some amazing people, I wrote a play which told the story of a dad whose daughter had died from epilepsy.

I was very fortunate that through my work, I was acquainted with people who could help me write the script and produce the show.

I knew that Karen's Wishes, was an important story and one which should be seen by all. When it was shown at the Mayfair Theatre in the West End of London in November 2010, it was a sell-out; I never imagined that it would be such a success.

Since Karen's death the family and I have been involved in lots of activities to raise awareness of what happened to her and the three people who die each day from epilepsy in the UK.

Ross Sheridan

Does surgery decrease the risk of SUDEP?

It is generally accepted that people with severe epilepsy are more at risk of SUDEP, so it would be reasonable to expect that people whose seizures are abolished by epilepsy surgery would have a reduced risk of SUDEP. The evidence however, is conflicting.

The most conclusive evidence comes from randomized controlled trials where people suitable for a treatment are randomly allocated to treatment or no treatment (frequently treatment with a placebo). It is ethically challenging to perform a prolonged study in which some people who are ideally suited for epilepsy surgery will be randomized to continuing medical treatment only. One short-term study randomized a group of 80 people with temporal lobe epilepsy thought suitable for surgery. Half had the centre's usual pre-surgical treatment (pre-surgical evaluation after one year on a waiting list), while those randomized to surgical treatment had the pre-surgical evaluation and subsequent surgery expedited (Wiebe et al. 2001). Only one person died during the year of follow-up after randomization– somebody in the waiting list group died of SUDEP. Despite the fact that SUDEP is more common in people with severe epilepsy, in any one time period only a small number of people will die from SUDEP; therefore statistical analysis is difficult.

Several studies have compared death rates in people who had epilepsy surgery and those who have not had surgery. Some in the non-surgical group may be waiting for surgical assessment or treatment, while others have been deemed not suitable for surgery; clearly these do not constitute the ideal control group. It is important to take the duration of follow-up into consideration as with longer follow-up, people are more likely to die. One group found that people who did not have surgery were more than twice as likely to die in the subsequent years as those who had surgery, and were four times as likely to die from SUDEP (Bell et al. 2010). A Swedish study also compared deaths in people who had surgery for epilepsy and those who only had pre-surgical evaluation; people who had surgery were slightly less likely to die than those who did not, and slightly fewer people died of SUDEP in the surgical group (Nilsson et al. 2003). Another study following people who had surgery between 1949 and 1988 and a control group found that more people who had surgery were seizure-free at two years, but that survival was no different in those who did and did not have surgery (Stavem & Guldvog 2005).

One study noted 11 deaths (six SUDEP) in 194 people who continued to have seizures after surgery, and no deaths in the 199 who became seizure-free (Sperling et al. 1999), and a similar study noted three deaths in 148 people who became seizure-free after epilepsy surgery, while eight of the 67 with continuing seizures died (Salanova, Markand & Worth 2002). The Swedish study, however, found no significant difference in SUDEP rate or overall mortality rate between those who were seizure-free at two years, and those who continued to have seizures (Nilsson et al.2003).

There are weaknesses in all studies which compare people who have surgery with those who do not, in particular when many of those who do not have surgery are not suitable for surgery. Various studies have suggested that people who are not suitable for epilepsy surgery are intrinsically different from those who are suitable, and may already have a higher risk of SUDEP (Ryvlin & Kahane 2003). Similarly, those who have a good outcome from surgery may have pre-existing differences from those who have a poor outcome (Jehi 2010). A study of the autonomic control of the heart rate in people who later had epilepsy surgery found that people with poor outcome of surgery are different in various measures of cardiac regulation from those with good outcome (Persson et al. 2005).

There have been fewer reports of death after vagal nerve stimulation (VNS) implantation. More than 1,800 people with VNS implantation for epilepsy were followed from implantation to death, deactivation, or the end of the study (Annegers et al. 2000). The rate of SUDEP was higher than the rate in antiepileptic drug trials; this is probably because VNS is only considered in people with severe epilepsy. The death rate for SUDEP was higher in the first two years than when the device had been working for two or more years.

In summary, this is an issue which requires further investigation.

Gail Bell
UCL Institute of Neurology, London, UK.

Mortality, epilepsy and neurological deficits

Developmental disabilities are associated with an increased risk of mortality (Forsgren et al. 1996, Day et al. 2005, Decoufle & Autry 2002). Such disabilities are also the single most important risk factor for death in people with epilepsy. This finding is seen repeatedly in studies of children and of adults in North America and Europe. Deaths occur for several distinct reasons including underlying neurodegenerative disorders, infectious complications from aspiration (whether in the context of a seizure or not), and of implanted medical devices such as shunts or feeding tubes, as well as due to other medical susceptibilities. Some deaths are clearly seizure-related involving suffocation or status epilepticus. In children, SUDEP appears to account for approximately 10% of deaths based on combined findings from 4 separate pediatric cohorts comprising over 2000 young people with epilepsy. Of the 69 deaths, almost all deaths occurred in children with neurodeficits (Berg et al. 2004, Camfield, Camfield & Veugelers 2002, Geerts et al. 2010, Nickels & Wirrell 2010); however, of the six documented SUDEP cases only 2 had neurodeficits. In a British study of children with epilepsy and intellectual disabilities, death rates were overall 16 times higher than expected from the general population, and 71% of deaths were epilepsy-related. The annual SUDEP incidence was 1/295 (Nashef et al. 1995).

By the same token, epilepsy is also a strong risk factor for death in people of all ages with developmental disabilities; however, the concept of SUDEP has been largely ignored. One large study found that, compared to the general population, people with epilepsy and disabilities were 64 times more likely to die with a cause of death identified as epilepsy, 124 times more likely to die with a cause of death identified as convulsion, and 5 times as likely to die with cause unknown (Day et al. 2005). As SUDEP was not an option in assigning cause of death, it is likely that SUDEP victims were placed into these categories thus making it impossible to assess the true burden of SUDEP in this neurologically impaired group. A separate Swedish study found that the presence of intellectual disability alone was associated with increased mortality in children although not in adults (Forsgren et al. 1996). In both children and adults and relative to the general population, the addition of epilepsy greatly increased mortality rates in people with intellectual disability and the further addition of cerebral palsy increased rates even further.

In theory, individuals with neurodeficits may be particularly prone to SUDEP by virtue of their brain injuries and conditions. While the mechanisms of SUDEP may be many and not fully understood at this time, the best evidence available implicates dysregulation of autonomic mechanisms including those involved in central cardiac and respiratory control. For patients with developmental disabilities in general, and for those with Dravet's syndrome in particular, where autonomic dysfunction can be marked and risk of SUDEP probably higher, comprehensive study of multi-modal physiological seizure characteristics may not only help identify individual risk but may substantially contribute to our current understanding of mortality. SUDEP-prone patients typically have frequent, treatment-refractory generalized tonic-clonic seizures; such seizures can produce profound autonomic dysfunction. In determining individual risk, recent evidence (Bateman, Spitz & Seyal 2010, Lhatoo et al. 2010) points to the value of studying electro-clinical seizure characteristics including oxygenation, capnography, EKG and EEG – parameters best studied in the epilepsy monitoring unit. Although many of these patients may not necessarily be surgical candidates, these investigations are still needed to identify susceptibility to autonomic dysfunction and hence risk for SUDEP. They should be performed when an increased risk is suspected.

In summary, although the pediatric cohorts reveal a high mortality rate in children with epilepsy who have neurodeficits, only about 10% of the deaths appear to be consistent with SUDEP. The risk may be greater in older patients; however, the available information does not explicitly address this issue effectively. From a pragmatic perspective, anyone with neurodeficit and epilepsy should be considered as especially vulnerable to mortality from a number of causes, many preventable such as accidents and drowning. To the extent that simple measure such as night time monitoring and reasonable supervision can prevent deaths from a variety of causes, these measures are reasonable and may contribute to a reduction in the risk of SUDEP although solid data are currently lacking on that point. Autonomic investigations should be considered when appropriate.

Anne T. Berg
Research Professor in Pediatrics
Children's Memorial Hospital, Chicago, IL, USA.

Samden D. Lhatoo
Professor of Neurology
University Hospitals Case Medical Center, Cleveland, OH, USA.

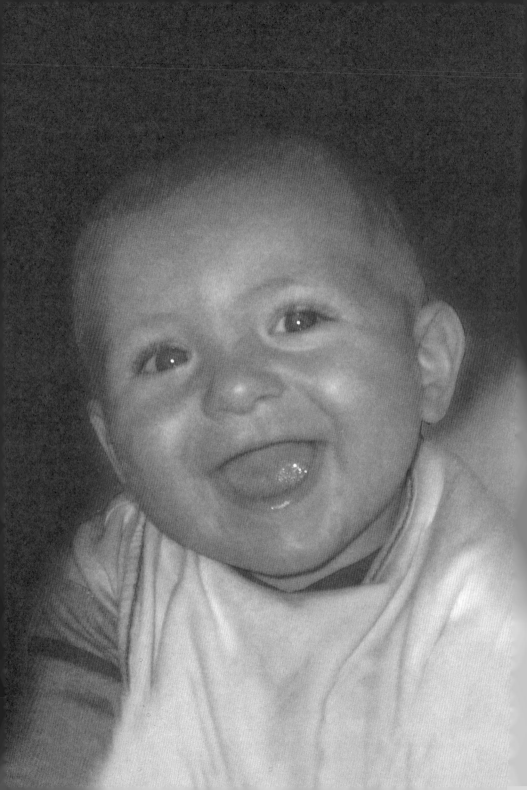

Rylee

October 2, 2007 we awoke to find that our two and a half year old son, Rylee, had passed away in the middle of the night. We called 911.

The police, ambulance, fire department and coroner arrived. I cannot tell you how many people were in our house, or how many times we had to recount our story. The police asked why our seizure alarm did not go off. I did not know. We had heard nothing on either the baby monitor or the alarm. I asked the coroner to consider SUDEP as a possible cause of death having learnt, through my own research on the internet, of its under reporting on death certificates. No doctor had mentioned SUDEP to me. Due to Rylee's age, I did not view him as a candidate. I never thought it would happen to us.

When the police left, I realized they had removed some items from the house (bedding, alarm, baby monitor and medication). This felt like a violation and added further distress as the requirements of an investigation were not explained to me.

While Rylee was alive, we made numerous trips to different emergency rooms. He suffered from 4 different types of seizures, was having about 2 grand mal seizures per day and was on 3 different medications. Doctors would ask if we wanted our son admitted and what tests we wanted run. I felt terrified; the medical professionals did not seem to know what to do with us and how to help manage our son's epilepsy. I became consumed with trying to learn as much as I could to try and advocate for my son.

SUDEP was listed as the cause of death. But, we had to wait 28 months to get the autopsy report as deaths of children under 5 must first undergo Paediatric Death Review Committee investigation prior to releasing results to the family.

In retrospect, I would advise people to get as much information as they can – to push for specialists and appropriate testing. Rylee was labelled by the paediatric neurologist as having severe epilepsy, but the doctor neither mentioned SUDEP nor referred us to an epileptologist.

I wonder now, what justifies a referral to this kind of specialist? I would strongly suggest that persons with epilepsy and their families educate themselves on all things related to epilepsy, ask questions, demand needs be met and, above all, do not give up.

Alaine Morrison

SUDEP and the post mortem

When someone close to us dies it is difficult to accept the need for a post mortem examination. Such examinations are almost always required when the death is sudden and unexpected; post mortems fall under the jurisdiction of the coroner to establish the cause. If epilepsy deaths are witnessed, information may be available as to whether a seizure took place. If the death is unwitnessed, for example occurring at night time or in the bathroom, there is less information for the pathologist and the possible modes of death are wider. The main categories of epilepsy-related death are: as a result of accident during a seizure (which includes head injury or drowning); as a result of a prolonged seizure (status epilepticus); aspiration during a seizure; and SUDEP. The post mortem can also exclude other natural causes of sudden death such as coronary artery disease, or a pulmonary embolus.

SUDEP is a negative post mortem where a cause of death is not found despite thorough organ examination and toxicology analysis. Establishing this category allows cases, which fit a pattern, to be grouped together and identified. The 'U' in SUDEP could equally stand for 'unexplained'; as we are still at the stage of 'hypothesis generation' (Tomson, Nashef & Ryvlin 2008). Epidemiological studies and current research support the notion that SUDEP is an ictal event and that cardiac, pulmonary or autonomic dysfunction concurrent with a seizure are the main mechanistic contenders. SUDEP is also likely to be multifactorial, with different causal mechanisms contributing in each case.

To understand what causes SUDEP, which is one step towards its prevention, 'global action' is required (Lathers 2009) with multidisciplinary team work including pathologists. Recognition of SUDEP was one of the main obstacles prior to the UK National Sentinel Audit (Hanna et al. 2002). Guidelines for best practice in epilepsy deaths were subsequently issued by the Royal College of Pathologists (2005). A national confidential enquiry (Lucas et al. 2006) into the coroners' autopsy, however, continued to single out post mortem examinations in epilepsy deaths as an area of specific concern, including the brain examination. This suggests that the practice is still not perfect.

The Royal College of Pathologists recommends that best practice in SUDEP is retention of the whole brain with fixation and thorough neuropathological examination including sampling of specific regions for microscopic examination, known to be vulnerable to alteration in patients with epilepsy. Alternatives are given as second and third best practice which include short fixation of the brain and/or regional brain sampling. We know that microscopic abnormalities (that cannot be seen with the naked eye or with MRI during life) can both cause seizures and directly or indirectly be a result of them. If the brain is examined only in the mortuary and returned directly to the body it is highly likely that such abnormalities will be missed and information lost.

What are the reasons for 'opting out' of best practice recommendations for SUDEP post mortems? Probably several: relatives reluctance for organ or tissue retention; changes in coroners' attitudes in the wake of Human Tissue Authority legislation; limitations on resources to fund a full examination; logistical problems in accessing a specialist neuropathological opinion; and the length of the neuropathological examination which can take several weeks. There are threats that this situation may get worse in the current era of financial cuts with proposals for an MRI or verbal autopsy as a substitute for anatomical dissection.

There are many arguments for continued retention and histological examination of the brain and other organs in SUDEP in addition to accuracy of the death certificate. As highlighted in a recent report from the American Epilepsy Society (So et al. 2009) there is great need for basic and clinical research in SUDEP which includes morphological, molecular, and biochemical studies of organs. These studies need to be carried out in centres which have gathered a large number of cases in order to provide meaningful information. In the UK at present there is no recognized epilepsy brain bank as a central point for tissue collection. Brain banks currently operating in the UK function as an excellent resource for research into neurodegenerative diseases, such as Alzheimer's disease. Similar strategies for SUDEP could link tissue based studies with clinical, epidemiological, and genetic data.

Central to any success in SUDEP research is the willing participation of bereaved relatives. Society's perception of a post mortem needs to change, not just as a morbid necessity but for positive gain. A brain donated to a bank or collection is as securely maintained and valued as a museum piece, which in some way lives on through research and collectively contributes to the study of the science behind the unexplained.

Maria Thom
UCL Institute of Neurology, London, UK.

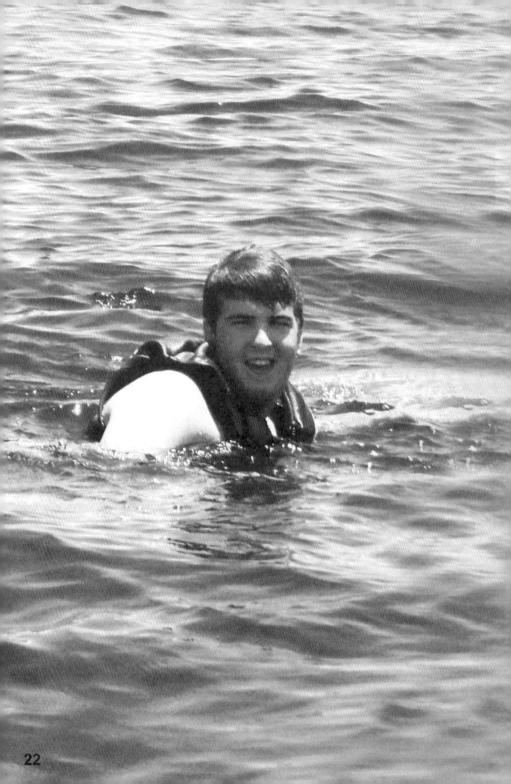

Eric

At 5am, on March 28, 2006, my wife and I woke to a loud crash. Running to our 16 year old son's room we found him on the floor, wedged between his bed and the nightstand, his lips blue and teeth clenched. He was having a seizure. This was new. Doctors said it might be a one-time event. His second seizure occurred 3 weeks later, then another one 3 days after that. Clearly this was not a one-time event.

We plunged into this, seeking as much information as we could and took him to the Mayo Clinic for a battery of tests. We were told that Eric could lead a long and normal life with epilepsy; there were only 2 areas of concern. Firstly, having a seizure in a dangerous situation (driving, swimming, rock climbing), and secondly, status epilepticus. We learned the harsh realities of epilepsy – there's no test to show that you have it, and no test to show that you're cured. You take meds and hope the seizures go away. SUDEP was never raised. Over time the doctors found a mix of meds that seemed to work and after 18 months the seizures appeared to be under control. For the most part they were infrequent and mild. For Eric, they always happened when he was sleeping, and they always woke us up.

On July 9, 2009, I awoke and went into Eric's room to check him as I did every morning. I noticed he was lying half on his bed, half on the floor. The dog was next to him. Eric had died in the middle of the night, on his mother's and brother's birthday.

Over the ensuing weeks I tried to cope with the loss of my son, to be there for his brother and mother, and to make some sense of it all. I worked with the coroner to find the cause of death. Toxicology reports indicated his meds were in the therapeutic range. While reading an article about epilepsy it hit me: Eric had died from SUDEP. I told the coroner that unless he could prove otherwise, I wanted Eric's death recorded as SUDEP. *As a father, I had to tell the coroner my son's cause of death*. When I explained SUDEP to him he said 'oh, we've had 3 or 4 similar cases in the past year'. Clearly, SUDEP is vastly under reported.

I expressed my frustration about the lack of SUDEP awareness to my primary physician, an ER doctor, also involved in Eric's treatment. He replied that he didn't know about SUDEP until I raised it. Comparing SUDEP with SIDS was interesting and frustrating – they are similar, striking seemingly healthy people, leaving no evidence after the fact, and there is nothing that can be done to prevent them. SIDS is widely known, while most doctors who are not neurologists have never heard of SUDEP. Yet in the US, SUDEP kills twice as many people as SIDS.

If I had been made aware of SUDEP could I have saved Eric's life? Possibly yes, possibly no. But without being told I wasn't given the chance.

It all starts with awareness.

Steve Wulchin

SUDEP: the need for standardized certification

When tabling SUDEP with governments and health services, hard data on numbers of SUDEP deaths can be powerful information to drive change towards reducing SUDEP.

However, accurately determining the number of SUDEP deaths is commonly hampered by various factors. Despite SUDEP being clearly defined, low rates of use of the term SUDEP on post mortem reports have been noted in a number of studies (Schraeder et al. 2006, 2009, Hanna et al. 2002). In a national survey of coroners and pathologists in the USA, with over 500 respondents, 84% of pathologists who responded acknowledged that they considered SUDEP a valid diagnosis if no cause of death was found at autopsy, but only 23% of these actually used the term SUDEP in more than half of cases where criteria for SUDEP were met (Schraeder et al. 2006).

SUDEP is not always a phenomenon that is *unexplained*, but rather *unexpected*. When the post mortem examination shows evidence of a recent seizure (such as tongue biting) or when there is evidence of asphyxia or suffocation (usually arising in the context of a seizure due to failure to correct body position in response to difficulties in breathing during or after the seizure), the death may certainly be explained as likely due to the adverse consequences of a seizure. Leading SUDEP authors argue that, although findings of asphyxia or suffocation or seizure may be noted at post mortem, these deaths should still be considered as SUDEP deaths as the definition of SUDEP encompasses unexpected death in a seizure (which may be related to cardiac or respiratory factors in the peri-seizure phase) and that it is unhelpful to separate out deaths with post mortem findings of seizure or asphyxia or suffocation (not least because the absence of these findings at post mortem does not exclude these as having happened and caused death) (Nashef & Ryvlin 2009).

Other factors that impact on understanding the incidence of SUDEP include consistency of terminology in recording epilepsy-related deaths on death certificates (Hanna et al. 2002), subsequent coding of cause of death by national statistics offices, practice in reporting of deaths to the coroner, actions of the coroner in deciding further examinations, completeness of post mortem investigation, access to these sources of information retrospectively by those researching SUDEP, and the availability of prospective data capture systems. In addition, variations in the laws of different countries may impact on the approach to investigation of sudden deaths in people with epilepsy.

In Australia, the Queensland Paediatric Epilepsy Network carried out a retrospective review of all epilepsy-related deaths in young people during a five-year period, using the Queensland Child Death Register that captures mortality data from both coronial and non-coronial Queensland-registered deaths of young people under the age of 18 years.

The study identified over sixty young people with epilepsy who had died in the five-year period, with reference to epilepsy or a similar term (e.g. seizures, convulsions) on the death certificate (two-thirds of deaths) or having the death referred to the coroner (one third of deaths). There was considerable inconsistency in the terminology used to record deaths from epilepsy on death certificates.

Although around a third of all deaths in young people with epilepsy were sudden, the term SUDEP was only used as the final post mortem diagnosis in around a third of the sudden deaths that had post mortem diagnosis available. In the majority of sudden deaths, the circumstances of death would have met the criteria for SUDEP or 'possible SUDEP' (Annegers & Coan 1999) (where post mortem investigations were not completed to allow criteria for SUDEP to be met, but all other factors were consistent). Instead of SUDEP, other diagnoses such as 'epilepsy', 'aspiration due to epilepsy', 'seizure' and 'respiratory failure due to epilepsy' were commonly found where SUDEP or 'possible SUDEP' would have been appropriate.

Data from this retrospective review indicate that we are a long way from accurately quantifying the number of SUDEP deaths currently occurring in Queensland (and by association in Australia), either from death certificate records or from post mortem diagnosis records. In order to be able to identify SUDEP deaths, agreed standards for certification of deaths in people with epilepsy are essential as are standardized approaches to reporting sudden deaths to coroners, standardized approaches to the post mortem investigations of these cases, and improved use of the term SUDEP on post mortem reports when criteria for SUDEP are met.

Kate Riney, Paediatric Neurologist & Epileptologist
University of Queensland
Mater Children's Hospital, QLD, Australia.

Damian Clark, Consultant Paediatric Neurologist
Women's and Children's Hospital Adelaide, SA, Australia.

SUDEP: medical data registers

The ultimate goal of all SUDEP research is to prevent death. The development of preventative strategies requires a better understanding of SUDEP, by comparing people who die from SUDEP to living people with epilepsy, and people with epilepsy who die of other causes. As retrospective reviews of SUDEP cases may limit the extent of data collection, many current research initiatives are employing medical data registries.

A medical data registry is a systematic collection of clearly defined health and demographic data for people with a certain health condition. Data can be collected from several sources and collated in one large database. Registries may include collection of biological samples, such as blood or tissue, for scientific study.

There are several approaches to the use of a registry for the study of SUDEP. One strategy is to continuously collect data on a large number of people with epilepsy and their condition over time. This prospective method has the advantage of providing more targeted, reliable data, as it does not rely upon memory or dated medical reports. It also allows for comparison of characteristics between living people with epilepsy and those dying from SUDEP or other causes. The disadvantage to this approach is that to ensure enough cases of SUDEP are available for meaningful study, a very large number of people with epilepsy need to be followed for many years, at considerable financial cost. It is hoped that new initiatives from research funding agencies will recognize the need for high quality prospective data collection and that funding will become available for such a large scale project.

A modification of this approach is to limit the collection of data to people with epilepsy who are already considered to be at higher risk of SUDEP, such as those with frequent generalized tonic-clonic seizures. This approach may be more cost effective and more likely to capture greater SUDEP cases for meaningful research, however, it disregards SUDEP cases of people with epilepsy at lower risk, who also require study. Another tactic is to search existing medical data registries for cases of SUDEP; however, few registries contain adequate information about people with epilepsy and their deaths.

A further method is to systematically collect information about SUDEP deaths as they occur. This approach may be the most economical; however, other sources must be used to obtain data about people with epilepsy for comparison. To date, most research has utilized this approach. In France, Dr. Marie-Christine Picot has established a network of neurologists, the French Epilepsy Mortality Surveillance Network, to systematically report deaths of people with epilepsy and case details, following family consent, to a central registry. In the UK, the SUDEP Research Initiative, a collaboration between King's College, London and Epilepsy Bereaved, is working to establish a SUDEP registry of deaths to be populated by health professionals and bereaved families. In Canada, we are developing a registry for SUDEP deaths in children. Prior to implementation, a survey will be sent to pediatricians across the country to both educate them to recognize SUDEP and gather information about SUDEP among Canadian children. A novel registry approach has been undertaken with the MORTality in Epilepsy Monitoring Unit Study (Mortemus). Dr Philippe Ryvlin of France, and colleagues worldwide, are collecting cases of deaths and near-deaths that occur during in-hospital video EEG monitoring. Given the level of intensive monitoring, this allows for very detailed information gathering around the time of a death or life threatening event.

All registry approaches rely on accurate identification of people with epilepsy and SUDEP deaths. Difficulties with case ascertainment are a recognized barrier to SUDEP research. In the UK, a 2002 audit of deaths of people with epilepsy demonstrated low autopsy rates and inconsistent use of the term epilepsy on death documentation (Hanna et al. 2002). A US survey of coroners and medical examiners also showed inconsistencies in the use of SUDEP as a final diagnosis (Schraeder et al. 2006). Education of healthcare providers, coroners, medical examiners and those affected by epilepsy is a critical step towards the development of effective, accurate and reliable registries. Once this can be achieved, these registries will constitute a vital tool in the race to understand SUDEP, to identify people with epilepsy at highest risk of SUDEP and to determine preventative strategies to reduce risk.

Elizabeth J. Donner
The Hospital for Sick Children, Toronto, Canada
Associate Professor, Faculty of Medicine (Pediatrics)
University of Toronto, Canada.

Mortality trends in general practice

The UK SUDEP Research Initiative, a collaboration between Epilepsy Bereaved and a team of researchers at King's College, University of London and King's College Hospital NHS Foundation Trust commissioned a study analyzing data from a large general practice population to look at trends in mortality (Ridsdale et al. 2011).

The UK General Practice Research Database (GPRD) contains information from patient records of a large population with a diagnosis of epilepsy and on antiepileptic medication. Since 2004 data has been more detailed as general practitioners have been rewarded for introducing an annual review for people with epilepsy and recording the percentage of patients who are seizure-free.

The research analyzed a cohort of people with epilepsy between 1993 and 2007. Research subjects included anyone diagnosed with epilepsy and prescribed antiepileptic medication. The study analyzed changes in the incidence, prevalence and mortality of epilepsy. Office for National Statistics data on deaths was also used to establish trends in mortality where epilepsy was coded as an underlying cause. A nested case-control study compared subjects with epilepsy who died with those who did not. We aimed to describe epilepsy incidence, prevalence, mortality and risk factors for death in epilepsy.

Prevalence of epilepsy increased from 9 per 1000 in 1993 to 12 per 1000 in 2007. The deaths in epilepsy rose by 31% in males and 39% in females between 1993 and 2005 at a time when mortality from all causes in the general population declined.

Patients who had alcohol problems were at almost three-fold increased risk, and risk in patients who had not collected their most recent anticonvulsant prescription for between 90 and 182 days was nearly doubled.

Having 'a history of injury' during the previous year increased risk by 40% and having treated depression increased risk by about the same amount. Patients who had been seizure-free in the previous 12 months had a 22% reduced risk of dying.

Since 2004 general practitioners have been remunerated for reporting on performance indicators for managing epilepsy, but so far they have not been remunerated for identifying risk factors for mortality, which are identified in the study. In the future we hope that general practitioner (GP) performance indicators will be linked to risk factors. We wish to develop the research to improve risk management in the community. For example, GPs could use computer software to flag up patients who have not collected their prescriptions for epilepsy medication.

The SUDEP Research Initiative has a programme of research. The next stage of the research is aimed at developing the potential of the national GP data to support risk management, and to analyze specific drug risks. The collaboration also supports the participation of bereaved relatives. A pilot study found that bereaved relatives were keen to participate in research and more detailed interviews are being conducted this year including a cohort of relatives where deaths were reported within the first year of diagnosis.

Leone Ridsdale
Professor of Neurology and General Practice
King's College, London, UK.

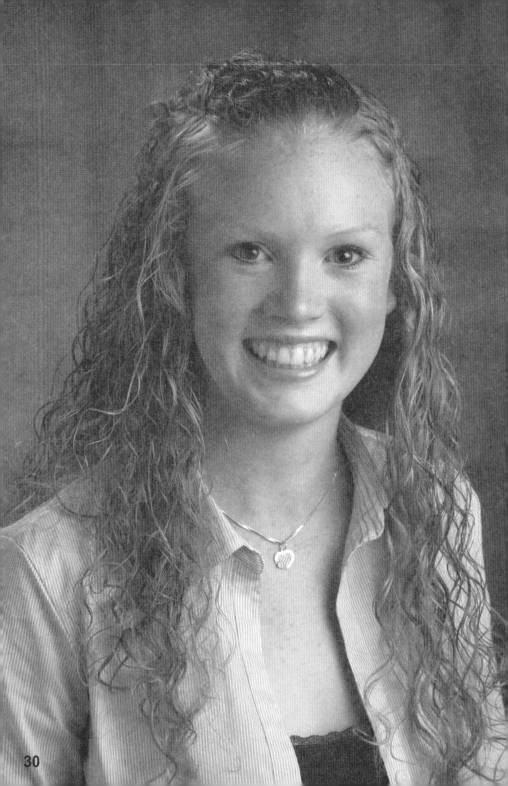

Jordan

Our precious Jordan, age 15, lived a short but very fulfilling life. In her resume, she describes herself as, 'an enthusiastic, responsible and eager person who loves sports and taking on new challenges.' She was a leader, mentor, friend, team player and was driven by her values and goals. Her positive approach to life was contagious and made people want to be with her. She was genuine, honest and open in all she did. She was strong and independent and made her own choices, even if they weren't popular. But most of all, Jordan was BRAVE!

Jordan suffered her first and only tonic-clonic seizure while trying out for a rep basketball team. One month later she was diagnosed with epilepsy, but was told this could be controlled with medication. The medication left Jordan feeling lethargic, slow, clumsy and in an overall depressive sort of state. Not the girl we were certainly used to. However, she continued on whilst experiencing almost weekly absence seizures, all of which were while playing sports.

Almost four months later, Jordan had her first neurologist appointment. Her medication was changed, due to the side effects, with the promise that the 'old her' would soon return. This did happen, gradually, over the following 10 weeks.

Jordan accepted her diagnosis with positivity. She never let it get her down, and she talked about it with everyone. She continued to play sports even through the tough times of new medications and seizures. She would say to the doctor, 'It's just a seizure, I'll get over it.'

We, and Jordan, spent a lot of time researching epilepsy on the internet and eventually learned of SUDEP from two lines of text in some hospital literature. It was classified as 'rare' and didn't seem to apply to Jordan.

Then the horrific day of November 2, 2010, only 12 months after her first seizure, we found Jordan face down in her bed, victim to SUDEP! One tonic-clonic seizure, a dozen absence seizures, and 6 months seizure-free, our precious daughter was stolen from us and our lives changed forever! We are left with the 'whys and how' and many unanswered questions.

Now we fight for more awareness as only through more awareness will the money for research come to answer all these questions, and hopefully save another family from the devastation ours must now endure.

Deb and Dave Fawcett

SUDEP and public policy

I have epilepsy myself, as well as another chronic condition, cerebral palsy. The cerebral palsy is part of my life, day in and day out; it never goes away. Epilepsy is qualitatively different. I often liken it to a thief in the night, because it creeps up unexpectedly (UK Parliamentary Debates 2010). I have nocturnal epilepsy which also means I am at risk of SUDEP.

From a UK policy perspective the National Outcomes Framework (NCHOD 2010) for health services prioritizes 'amenable mortality' and epilepsy is included in those conditions considered 'amenable'. Definitions of amenable mortality vary in international policy development, but the concept is aimed at flagging premature deaths related to conditions which can be controlled with timely and effective medical care and services, and the cooperation of the individual. It is a warning of 'potential shortcomings' and identifies the need for detailed analysis.

In the UK, the last detailed analysis of the national statistics was the National Audit of Epilepsy-Related Deaths (Hanna et al. 2002) which found that a significant number of deaths (42%) were potentially avoidable. Deaths were found in people who were not known to be seizure-free and many of these people had not accessed epilepsy services to enable better control. In policy terms the audit was instrumental in raising the profile of epilepsy with governments across the UK and an unprecedented series of national epilepsy policy initiatives followed including an annual epilepsy review by GPs, national clinical and pathology guidelines, and in Wales, a Commissioning Directive.

By 2011, national statistics reveal a small increase in the rate of reported epilepsy deaths. Premature deaths related to epilepsy accounted for 70,096 'lost years' between 2006 and 2008. Understanding these statistics is not straightforward. We know that implementation of national initiatives has been sporadic, but we also know that in the UK there has been heightened awareness of SUDEP amongst pathologists and coroners.

Monitoring of epilepsy deaths is critical to any strategy on amenable mortality. National registers which look beyond the death statistics to review clinical and other relevant data are urgently needed to improve understanding. Critical event monitoring as well as investigatory bodies such as the UK child death overview panels and coroners' inquests also have an important part to play.

International mortality league tables have been mooted but are likely to mislead policy makers because of differences in systems for investigating and reporting deaths, combined with the lack of understanding and application of SUDEP as a category of death.

Whilst the cause of SUDEP is not fully understood, a patient-centred preventative strategy focussing on seizure risk management that acknowledges the strong association between SUDEP and seizures, is in keeping with the aim to address the 'amenability' of deaths.

UK National guidelines recognise the importance of seizure-freedom and being aware of the dangers of night seizures and although they recommend that SUDEP be part of essential information to patients following diagnosis (Stokes et al. 2004), the sharing of such information is sporadic. I understand SUDEP from my work as a politician and not because I have ever been told about it as a person with epilepsy.

Attitudes towards epilepsy may continue to be responsible for the lack of attention to addressing epilepsy mortality. Research is critical in unlocking the cultural and service barriers to implementing risk reduction in epilepsy and to better understand the potential avoidability of deaths listed each year in mortality statistics.

Paul Maynard, Member of Parliament, House of Commons, UK.

Part 2.

facing the questions

The evolution of SUDEP research

From the 1950's to the 1990's, single SUDEP cases, as well as collections of multiple SUDEP cases (descriptive case series), were reported in the medical literature with increasing frequency. Many of the reports came from university-based epilepsy programs that cared for patients with medically resistant epilepsy. In that setting, the frequency of SUDEP was shown to be alarmingly high. SUDEP was reported to account for up to 60% of deaths that occurred in young adults with epilepsy. The risk of SUDEP over a one-year period in patients with uncontrolled epilepsy was calculated in different studies to range from one in every 100 to one in every 250 persons.

Because SUDEP can only be definitely diagnosed if autopsy shows no natural or accidental cause for the death (Nashef 1997), the importance of an autopsy series of SUDEP cases was recognized. Dr. Leestma (1989) published the clinical and autopsy results of a prospective series of SUDEP cases in Chicago, USA and this study is still one of few well planned studies that described autopsy findings in SUDEP. Following Dr. Leestma's study, collections of SUDEP cases were analyzed and reported with increasing frequency in Europe, Australia and North America. From these reports, we began to appreciate that the risk of SUDEP in persons with uncontrolled seizures that have not responded to medications is much higher than the risk in persons with well-controlled epilepsy. Moreover, case-control studies provided some consistent findings across different studies. The studies consistently identified generalized tonic-clonic seizures ('grand mal' convulsions) as a major risk for SUDEP. This is not to say that other types of seizures, such as complex focal seizures without convulsion, do not carry SUDEP risk. However, the risk is smaller. In fact, the SUDEP risk in some seizure-types such as absence ('petit mal') seizures is negligible. Population-based studies, which studied all epilepsy persons and not just intractable epilepsy persons, also showed that SUDEP risk in general is reassuringly low.

Lathers and Schraeder (1990) published the first book on SUDEP, which discussed both clinical and experimental data known about SUDEP up to that point. A SUDEP symposium was also published in 1997, which discussed key issues in SUDEP definition, epidemiology, pathogenic mechanisms, and education and counselling issues (Nashef, Annegers & Brown 1997). Since then, more animal models of SUDEP have been developed and studied, some to investigate respiratory mechanisms in SUDEP, and others to assess autonomic and genetic bases that potentially underlie SUDEP. Lay organizations were established with a specific focus on SUDEP issues, including counselling of patients and their families about SUDEP risk, education of health care providers about SUDEP and its mitigation, and support of bereaved families of SUDEP victims. Epilepsy Bereaved of UK is one such pioneer organization, and there are now several other such organizations around the world. In 2004, the National Institute for Clinical Excellence in the UK emphasized the need for early and tailored counselling of patients and families regarding SUDEP risks (Stokes et al. 2004).

More recently in 2007, major epilepsy organizations in the US, namely American Epilepsy Society (AES), Epilepsy Foundation (EF) and Citizens United for Epilepsy (CURE) supported the establishment of the AES-EF Joint SUDEP Task Force. The assessment and recommendations of the Task Force were published in 2008 (So et al. 2009). Subsequently, the National Institute of Neurological Disorders and Stroke (NINDS) of the US convened a SUDEP workshop, the participants of which were national and international clinicians, researchers, patient advocates, ethics and legal experts, many of whom did not have prior work in SUDEP, but had experience and knowledge in disciplines related to SUDEP. The goal of the workshop was to derive guidance from a wide range of expertise on the directions of future SUDEP research. Currently, the American Academy of Neurology and the American Epilepsy Society are jointly developing guidelines on the clinical approach to SUDEP issues, including education and counselling of patients and care providers.

There is no doubt that SUDEP research and advocacy is picking up pace in different parts of the world. In my opinion, it would not be unrealistic to expect groundbreaking knowledge about SUDEP to surface over the next five to ten years.

Elson L. So
Professor of Neurology
Mayo Clinic College of Medicine, Rochester, MN, USA.

The conundrum of SUDEP

Two categories of disturbances of normal physiology have been implicated in SUDEP. The most common is seizure-related neurogenic cardiac rhythm disturbance; the other is neurogenic respiratory disturbance in the form of lung edema and apnea. These two types of seizure-related disturbances have been studied clinically and experimentally in efforts to define the mechanism(s) of SUDEP. In addition, the possible role of psychological stress has only recently been raised. Research over the past two decades has provided a remarkable increase in the amount of data but, unfortunately, an understanding of the mechanism(s) still eludes us. In essence, we remain in a state of ignorance, but with a greater data base.

Cardiac: The association of seizures with self limited, non fatal cardiac arrhythmias is well established. The most common of these is tachycardia in association with generalized tonic-clonic seizures. A less common observation is slowing of the heart rate (bradycardia) that on occasion devolves to brief cardiac arrest in association with temporal lobe or frontal lobe partial seizures. Long term electrocardiogram recording data from persons who subsequently succumbed to SUDEP show an ongoing disturbance of autonomic cardiac regulation as manifested by decreased ability to vary the heart rate in response to different circumstances, especially during non rapid eye movement (NREM) sleep. How these common, usually reversible, seizure-related cardiac changes may in some persons result in SUDEP is not known. Another possible factor is cardiac sodium channel disturbance associated with an abnormal *SCN5A* gene, raising the question of whether this genetic disturbance, if present in persons with epilepsy, increases the risk of seizure associated cardiac arrhythmias. Animal models demonstrate that seizure activity is associated with disturbances of autonomic innervation to the heart that can predispose to arrhythmias (Lathers & Schraeder 2011a, Herreros 2011).

Respiratory: Neurogenic acute respiratory disturbance is also viewed as a possible mechanism in SUDEP. Reversible pulmonary edema occurs occasionally in persons with severe generalized seizures, such as status epilepticus. Most victims of SUDEP have increased post mortem lung weights from increased lung fluid, a phenomenon that is considered to be neurogenic pulmonary edema. Animal models of respiratory changes have demonstrated that both acute pulmonary edema and central nervous system apnea can be induced by seizures. While the mechanism for respiratory arrest is not defined, recent clinical studies suggest that abnormally prolonged postictal generalized electroencephalographic (EEG) suppression (PGES), i.e, greater that 50 seconds, may lead to central apnea. Although this data on PGES may represent a new mechanistic insight and deserves further investigation, it is important not to dismiss the large body of data implicating cardiac dysfunction as a potential mechanism involved in SUDEP (Finsterer & Stollberger 2011, Lhatoo et al. 2010).

Psychological: Another mechanistic factor that has been mostly ignored and which may be contributory to SUDEP is emotional stress. Stress has a well established association with sudden death in persons with coronary artery disease and in those with a history of psychiatric disorders. Such deaths are associated with threat of loss of a close person, loss of status or self esteem, and threat of, or paradoxically, relief from personal danger. Having epilepsy is associated with ongoing psychological stresses. Examples are fear of embarrassment, loss of driving privileges, loss of employment, and concern about injury consequent to a seizure. More investigative work is needed in determining if psychological factors play a mechanistic role in SUDEP (Lathers & Schraeder 2006).

Summary: Data seem to suggest that the mechanism of SUDEP may be dependent upon individual susceptibility to one or a combination of factors. These may include: seizure-related central apnea and/or lung edema with respiratory death; seizure-related hypoxia plus acute pulmonary changes and systemic acidosis leading to a fatal arrhythmia; an inherited cardiac ion channelopathy combined with acute seizure-related cardiac autonomic disruption leading to a fatal arrhythmia. Added to the mix is the unknown of acute psychological stress. The mechanism(s) of SUDEP remain a mystery, but with a growing interest in investigating the mechanistic variables, there is reason to be optimistic that eventually it will be solved.

Paul L. Schraeder
Department of Neurology (emeritus)
Drexel University College of Medicine, Philadelphia, PA, USA.

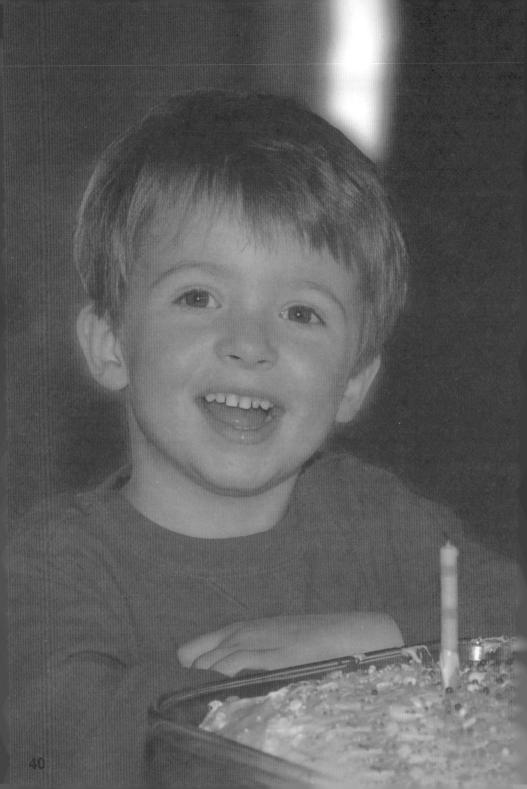

Henry

My son, Henry, was a beautiful, happy and healthy little boy. As a 3-year old he suffered from a few febrile seizures. His medical evaluation for these seizures revealed nothing and we soon learned that they are not uncommon in childhood. However, a few months after his 4th birthday, he had a seizure that was not associated with a fever. Before his epilepsy work-up was even complete and before he had a chance to become therapeutic on his medication, Henry died in his sleep from SUDEP.

A mere five weeks after our son's first epileptic seizure, he had died. It happened so fast. In addition to the horrific pain of losing my oldest son, I felt so blindsided. How could this have happened? He had great medical care. The odds were that he would grow out of this childhood epilepsy. And to think, I had a background in nursing and public health and still had no idea that epilepsy could be so devastating.

After months of anger and sadness, I discovered CURE (Citizens United for Research in Epilepsy). CURE was founded by parents of children with epilepsy who were frustrated by their inability to protect their children from the devastation of seizures and the side effects of medications. It was among some of these parents that I found understanding and through CURE that I found hope.

Since joining the CURE board, I have become more involved in advancing understanding around SUDEP. I have shared our story publicly to raise awareness of the need for research as well as the need for providers to discuss SUDEP with their patients. Our family also support CURE's SUDEP-focused grant program and has had the opportunity to fund innovative and exciting research.

I most enjoy working with other epilepsy organizations as well as clinicians, researchers and professionals from NIH (National Institutes of Health) and CDC (Center for Disease Control). While there is still such a long way to go, I am thankful for the growing US interest in SUDEP. This is most evidenced by more governmental funding being made available to advance research. Additionally, more epilepsy organizations are working together towards a common goal to fund research and advance provider and patient understanding and communication around SUDEP. It keeps me going to be part of these efforts.

Though I cannot bring Henry back, I hope for nothing more than to prevent others from having to suffer such a loss. I firmly believe that with persistence we can unravel the mysteries of SUDEP and put an end to the fear and anguish it causes.

Gardiner Lapham

Basic mechanisms of SUDEP: animal studies

Research consistently points at three main possible SUDEP mechanisms: autonomic dysfunction, respiratory compromise and cardiac arrhythmias.

Autonomic system and brain heart connections in SUDEP: Laboratory research has been vital to our improved understanding of SUDEP causes. Animal investigations show that overactivity and imbalance in the autonomic nervous system can cause wide fluctuations in blood pressure, inefficient cardiac function, and excessive airway secretions. External airway obstruction with pillows or prone sleeping position may lead to a fatal seizure outcome.

Still, what are the triggers setting off the cascade of events leading to SUDEP? Initial answers came from mouse models carrying human mutations for the often lethal cardiac arrhythmia, the long QT syndrome (LQTS). In 2009, researchers discovered that an ion channel gene, *KCNQ1*, responsible for the most common form of LQTS, can trigger potentially fatal fainting spells but can also cause epilepsy, putting patients at risk of sudden death (Goldman et al. 2009). Subsequently another candidate SUDEP gene, an epilepsy ion channel gene, *KCNA1*, was found to be important for normal function of both brain and heart (Glasscock et al. 2010). Mice deficient in *KCNA1* developed arrhythmias of the heart with the rhythm disturbances more severe during seizures. Most of the mice who lacked this channel gene died prematurely as a result of their frequent seizures and in close resemblance to the few reported witnessed instances of human SUDEP. Moreover, both *KCNQ1* and *KCNA1* are present in the vagus nerve that physically connects the heart and the brain, provides fibres to the throat and airways, and is critical in the regulation of the autonomic functions (Goldman et al. 2009, Glasscock et al. 2010). Interestingly, a cardiology laboratory has also verified that many episodes in individuals with confirmed LQTS are likely to be epileptic seizures rather than fainting spells (Johnson et al. 2009). These are important findings. It means that a seizure, and not just a fainting spell, could signify that a patient may have a heart rhythm disturbance and be at risk for sudden death.

The importance of the autonomic nervous system balanced function has been demonstrated in additional animal models; Sakamoto et al. (2008) reported an 8-10 fold increase in the vagal activity during seizures of a urethane/kainic acid rat model. Stimulation of the efferent vagus nerve applied externally or during seizures caused a collapse in the systemic blood pressure and impaired filling of the heart ventricles (Hotta et al. 2009). Stimulation of the sympathetic system that forms a functional counterpart to the vagus nerve led to improvement in arterial pressure but a simultaneous worsening in cardiac performance. The parasympathetic/vagal overactivity was also responsible for airway secretions that interfered with effective ventilation (Hotta, Koizumi & Stuart 2009). Therefore, defective function of the autonomic system can not only underlie epilepsy-related cardiac arrhythmias but compromise effective respiration especially during the seizures.

Respiratory compromise and SUDEP: DBA/2 mice provide another important clue for the possible mechanism of the impaired ventilation during seizures. The animals develop fatal respiratory arrest during generalized convulsive seizures and the susceptibility to ictally induced respiratory arrest appears linked to the changes in the expression of the serotonin (5-hydroxytryptamine or 5-HT) receptors that are part of a molecular system involved in seizures, breathing, arousal, and in sudden death in animal models and humans (Buchanan & Richerson 2010, Richerson & Buchanan 2011). Aberrations in the 5-HT neuronal firing seem to be critically involved in the ictal hypoventilation and in the depression of the ictal and postictal arousal (Richerson & Buchanan 2011). Interestingly, the risk for seizure-related sudden death appears to be minimized by giving animals a commonly used antidepressant compound acting as a 5-HT receptor agonist. This finding has important implications for future human research and for clinical practice (Uteshev et al. 2010).

Other molecular mechanisms: Genes in the adenosine receptor pathway are important for proper cardiac performance and respiration with an effect on seizures and SUDEP risk. Recent experiments showed that stimulation of the adenosine receptors may lower seizure threshold and lead to seizure-related death (Fukuda et al. 2011). Conversely administration of an adenosine receptor antagonist, caffeine, increased animal survival (Shen, Li & Boison 2010).

The recent discoveries of the genes and molecular systems involved in epilepsy, heart arrhythmias, and respiration are an important milestone. Brain regions involved in seizure generation are extensively linked with the brain stem where the respiratory centres are intimately connected with the cardiac autonomic nuclei. Hence, seizure induced respiratory or cardiac compromise could trigger a lethal interaction between the seizure, impaired ventilation, lack of arousal, and cardiac arrhythmias resulting in SUDEP.

Alica M. Goldman
Assistant Professor of Neurology
Baylor College of Medicine, Houston, Texas, USA.

Basic mechanisms of SUDEP: human studies

The clinical research in humans has paralleled the investigations in animals when exploring the chief theories of SUDEP biology. Additionally, there have been analyses of possible environmental factors contributing to SUDEP (Terra et al. 2011).

Respiratory compromise in SUDEP: Seizure-related ictal oxygen desaturation has been observed in epilepsy patients (Bateman, Li & Seyal 2008) and in SUDEP (Bateman, Spitz & Seyal 2010). The analysis of 61 seizures in 10 patients with temporal lobe epilepsy revealed that the onset of apnea was significantly linked to the contralateral seizure spread. These findings identified a patient group at high risk for seizure-related respiratory compromise and possibly SUDEP (Seyal & Bateman 2009). Another investigation translated the results obtained in the DBA/2 mouse model (Uteshev et al. 2010) and examined the influence of the serotonin reuptake inhibitor (SSRI) class of antidepressants on ictal desaturation in epilepsy patients. The authors found decreased severity in the ictal oxygen desaturation in partial seizures of patients chronically exposed to the SSRIs compared to the subjects not taking the antidepressant preparations. There was no definite protective effect of the SSRIs on ventilation in generalized seizures (Bateman et al. 2010).

Cardiac arrhythmias in SUDEP: The animal research has major influence on the investigations in patients; Tu et al. (2011) analyzed 68 post mortem SUDEP samples for mutations in the three most common LQT genes, *KCNQ1*, *KCNH2*, and *SCN5A*. The authors found several genetic variations that have been previously identified in LQTS patients (Tu et al. 2011). The study design did not allow for proof of causality. However, it underscored the importance of a focused and systematic research on genomic variation in a candidate gene set in well-characterized SUDEP cases in our quest for defining the SUDEP molecular risk factors.

Clinical markers of autonomic function: As evidenced by animal and clinical studies impaired autonomic control plays a key role in epilepsy-related cardiac arrhythmias, and heart rate variability was explored as a potential marker of cardiac/autonomic function. The epilepsy patients seem to consistently show decreased heart rate variability (HRV) compared to healthy individuals (Mukherjee et al. 2009, Toth et al. 2010, Yildiz et al. 2011). Moreover, HRV was influenced by epilepsy syndrome and was found to fluctuate depending on the drugs used to treat seizures (Delogu et al. 2011, Yildiz et al. 2011). These results together with the discoveries of the role of LQT genes in epilepsy and

SUDEP underscore the importance of routine electrocardiogram (ECG) in the screening of cardiac functions in the patients with epilepsy before and during therapy with antiepileptic medications.

Electrocerebral shutdown hypothesis is based on the observations of the severe depression of electrocerebral activity on the electroencephalogram (EEG) following a seizure that can, in some patients, lead to SUDEP. The data stems from patients that were monitored in the epilepsy monitoring units (Lhatoo et al. 2010, Tao et al. 2010). The ECG recording and the motion artifact on the EEG tracing indicated ongoing cardiac and respiratory efforts following the onset of EEG depression and before the terminal cessation of all functions. Unfortunately, the ECG data are limited and there is no pulse oximetry as a minimal objective measurement of the ventilation. Therefore, there is no definite clarity about the complex interplay between the brain, heart, and respiration.

Environmental factors in epilepsy and SUDEP: Limited research data suggest that polyunsaturated fatty acids (PUFAs) found in olive oil and fish may have beneficial impact on neural and cardiovascular function (Terra et al. 2011). However, the results are currently insufficient for drawing more definite conclusions or recommendations.

The acronym SUDEP is used variably to stand for sudden unexplained death in epilepsy vs. sudden unexpected death in epilepsy. The strides in science are gradually eliminating the term 'unexplained' although the event still remains 'unexpected'. We have defined the first set of genetic risk factors and made progress in elucidating some of the critical mechanisms behind the autonomic dysfunction and cardio-respiratory compromise in SUDEP. The discoveries in the basic and in the human research are driving the development of patient at risk screening protocols (EKG, pulse oximetry, genetic analysis) and preventative measures (anti-arrhythmic medications, cardiac defibrillators or pacemakers, supplemental oxygen, SSRI class of antidepressants). Much remains obscure. However, a systematic collection of tissue samples, generously donated by epilepsy patients and SUDEP victims, is invaluable in promoting the legacy of our patients in the quest for prevention and cure of this presently lethal epilepsy outcome.

Alica M. Goldman
Assistant Professor of Neurology
Baylor College of Medicine, Houston, Texas, USA.

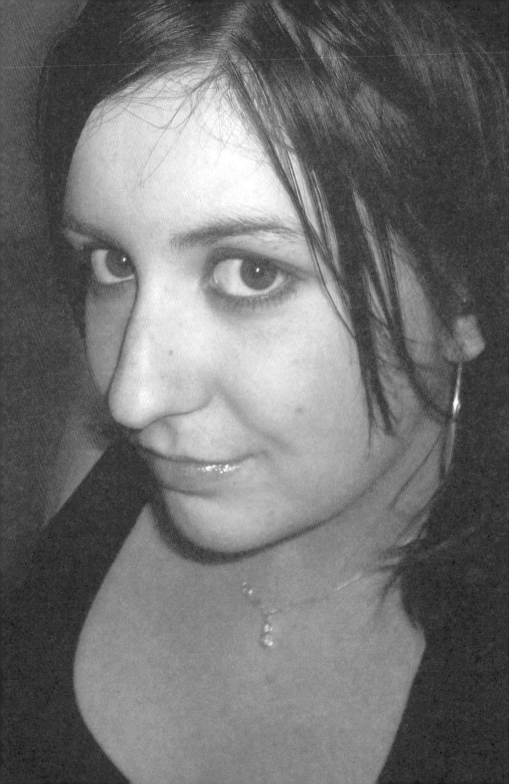

Ebony

Ebony or Ebz as she was known to her friends, passed away in her bedroom on Sunday, 16th May 2010 — three weeks after we celebrated her 21st birthday. We never suspected that Ebony could be having seizures.

She had recently started her dream position working for a recruiting company in the mining industry. Her employers were very impressed by her work and work ethic, telling me that she was made for the position. She enjoyed the independence that working gave her. Ebony had plans – the company's head office is in Sweden, and she was so hopeful to go there and see their base. She had also booked flights to Perth to surprise her friend for her 21st birthday.

The last twelve months or so before her passing away, Eb was chronically tired and constantly complained of headaches. We ensured Eb had plenty of water to drink and we monitored her heart rate and blood pressure, which was elevated. Ebony had a few presentations to the local emergency department, as at times she complained her heart was pounding through her chest. On numerous occasions Eb would say that her head felt funny, so again we monitored her blood pressure and pondering solutions we purchased a glucometer to monitor her blood glucose level, as we have diabetes in our family. Her blood glucose level was within normal limits.

Our local GP sent Ebony for tests which included an echocardiogram and ECG, along with several blood tests, none of which provided any answers. As a child Eb was a chronic snorer and suffered chronic tonsillitis, so the GP sent her for sleep studies; again no answers were found. He then decided to have an EEG performed. Unfortunately this was booked for the week after she had passed.

As Ebony passed away at home with no suspicious circumstances her death was automatically referred to the coroner. Initially no cause of death could be determined, and toxicology reports were negative for alcohol and drugs. This resulted in the need for a closer examination of her brain in an attempt to find a cause of death. The medical examiner informed us that her brain had travelled to the best pathologists in Australia with results showing, and unbeknown to us, that Ebony had suffered previous frontal lobe seizures, therefore a cause of death was recorded as epilepsy.

The day of her funeral, friends came from all over Australia, which to us was a reflection of the type of person she was. Ebony's favourite colour was purple, ironically the colour that represents epilepsy.

Ebony was a true and very honest person, if you were her friend you were a friend no matter what. She was her sister's protector whom she totally adored. Her last facebook status said 'life is sweet'.

Unfortunately for us, left to carry on without her, time was not on her side.

Debbie Johnson

SUDEP and matters of the heart

SUDEP is likely to have a variety of causes. One of them may involve dysfunction of the heart due to cardiac arrhythmia which could lead to insufficient blood circulation and fatal decrease of oxygen supply. Bradycardia and asystole are well known seizure-related phenomena. In contrast, life-threatening ventricular tachyarrhythmias have been hypothesized for decades as a potential cause of SUDEP, but convincing clinical evidence has been lacking.

There are a number of established risk factors of sudden cardiac death which increase the susceptibility to ventricular tachyarrhythmias (Surges et al. 2009, 2010). One important risk factor appears to be pathological cardiac repolarization. Cardiac repolarization is the phase of the cardiac cycle during which the electrical potential of heart muscle cells returns from excitation to the resting condition. The QT interval is an ECG indicator of cardiac repolarization. Prolongation of the QT interval above normal limits (which depend on age, gender and actual heart rate) is a well characterized risk factor for sudden cardiac death. Genetic forms, known as long QT syndromes, are due to mutation in various ionic channels responsible for the electrical properties of the heart. Pathological QT prolongation is also seen with the use of drugs such as some antibiotics and antidepressants. A decade ago, a genetic form of abnormally short QT interval, also due to mutations in cardiac ionic channels, has been discovered. People with short QT syndrome display QT intervals below normal limits, suffer from syncope due to atrial fibrillation, ventricular tachycardia and fibrillation, and have a high risk of sudden cardiac death. QT dispersion is another measure of cardiac repolarization. It is the difference between the longest and shortest QT interval on an ECG recording and reflects the regional heterogeneity of cardiac repolarization. Values above 50-60 ms have been shown to increase the risk of sudden cardiac death in apparently healthy people and in other medical conditions.

Features of cardiac repolarization have recently been investigated in people with chronic epilepsy. Abnormal QT dispersion was seen in up to one third of people with focal epilepsy. Changes of QT interval during seizures have also been investigated recently. Prolongation of QT interval was found in up to 12% of people with focal epilepsy. Transient abnormal shortening of QT interval has been observed to occur with almost every convulsive seizure in people with temporal lobe epilepsy. Antiepileptic drugs seem to have only minor effects on the QT interval. Valproate has no direct action on cardiac repolarization, but can enhance QT prolongation of co-administered drugs which themselves lengthen QT interval and which are metabolized by specific liver enzymes (inhibited by valproate). In contrast, rufinamide, primidone and carbamazepine have been reported to shorten QT interval. To date, the clinical importance of acquired QT shortening is unclear and is currently under investigation.

Abnormalities of cardiac repolarization are common in people with chronic epilepsy. The question is, however, whether these abnormalities are benign or whether they increase the risk for sudden cardiac death as one plausible cause for SUDEP. In a recent case report, ventricular tachycardia and fibrillation were described shortly after a convulsive attack in a person with epilepsy. This woman was successfully resuscitated, and subsequent cardiological investigations have not shown any underlying cardiac disease, suggesting that seizure-related alterations of cardiac excitability may have facilitated the life-threatening ventricular tachyarrhythmia in this person.

In summary, there is evidence that abnormal cardiac repolarization and ventricular tachyarrhythmia could cause sudden death in some people with epilepsy. The most important question is whether arrhythmia-related SUDEP can be predicted and prevented. To date, it is difficult to say who would benefit from preventive measures, which actions to be taken and at what time point. Potential measures to reduce the risk or to prevent SUDEP could, however, include anti-arrhythmic medication (such as beta-blockers which are used in some forms of long QT syndrome) and implantation of a defibrillator device (to stop ventricular tachycardia). Current research focuses on the risk factors and mechanisms leading to epilepsy-related abnormalities in cardiac repolarization. Collaborative multi-centre efforts are needed to find out whether these ECG features are helpful to identify people at higher risk for SUDEP and to develop strategies to prevent SUDEP due to cardiac arrhythmia.

Rainer Surges
Department of Epileptology
University Clinics, Bonn, Germany.

SUDEP: heart and brain link

SUDEP is the most common cause of epilepsy-related death and responsible for about 150 Australian deaths each year yet the underlying cause has remained a mystery. SUDEP is the term applied to sudden death occurring in a person with epilepsy for no apparent reason. When such a death occurs and all other possible causes of death are excluded, SUDEP is usually attributed as the cause of death. Several studies have proven that cardiac and respiratory problems associated with recurring seizures could be factors contributing to the cause of SUDEP. The most commonly suggested cause is a fatal abnormal heart rhythm consequently leading to the sudden death of a person with epilepsy. Recently research revealed SUDEP is caused by DNA changes in genes involved in how the heart cells regulate sodium, potassium and calcium through structures called ion channels.

We discovered the presence of DNA changes in cardiac ion channels responsible for the potentially fatal heart disorder known as familial Long QT syndrome (Tu et al. 2010). Familial Long QT syndrome is caused by mutations in more than 10 genes and eight of these can interfere with the ion channel of cell membranes and disrupt their ability to regulate electrical activity in our body. This disruption of the ion channels can lead to abnormal, life-threatening heart rhythms consequently leading to sudden death.

My research team identified a group of people with epilepsy in Sydney, Australia who died from a sudden unexpected death between 1993 to 2009. A total of 68 SUDEP cases were found and 40 cases (62%) were taking antiepileptic drug therapy and 64 cases (94%) were unwitnessed events, were in good health within 24h of discovery and found deceased in bed. Post mortem blood samples for cases of SUDEP were thoroughly evaluated for DNA changes in the three most common Long QT syndrome genes (*KCNQ1, KCNH2 (HERG), SCN5A*). Interestingly, of the 48 cases that could be analyzed DNA changes were present in six (13%) cases.

These findings demonstrate DNA changes that disrupt the ion channels play a role in sudden death in people with epilepsy. However, we were unable to review medical histories to look at a family history of sudden death, epilepsy and/or Long QT syndrome so it remains to be determined whether these changes are the genetic cause or an accompanying risk factor. While the findings are a major first step in understanding the cause of SUDEP more research is needed to determine the exact role these genetic changes play.

Subsequent studies on these SUDEP cases revealed DNA changes in other ion channels present in both the heart and brain, indicating an additional causal link in the sudden death of a person with epilepsy.

Sudden unexpected death in epilepsy occurs mainly in young people so these findings could have a huge impact in saving lives through early diagnosis. The ultimate goal will be to use genetic screening of patients with epilepsy to identify these gene mutations that could increase the risk of sudden unexpected death.

Emily Tu, Richard D. Bagnell, Johan Duflou & Christopher Semsarian
Molecular Cardiology
Centenary Institute, Newtown, NSW, Australia.

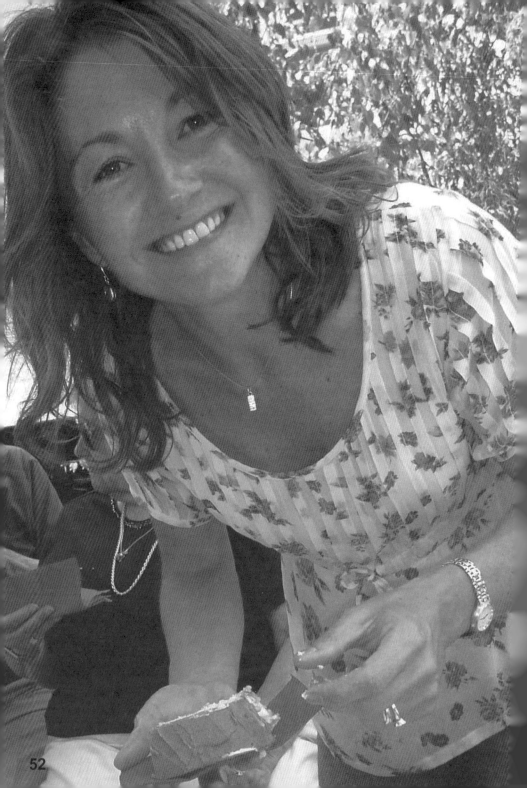

Kirsty

Kirsty was one of a pair. She has an identical twin sister– a mirror twin – a wonderful constant reminder. Kirsty's first episode of epilepsy was at the age of 18 (petit mal). Her visible symptoms were inattentiveness, hand gestures and occasional nonsensical language. These episodes occurred infrequently but due to their unusual nature, we sought medical advice. Kirsty was diagnosed with front temporal lobe epilepsy and, with medication, she would have nothing much to worry about.

Kirsty investigated brain surgery but was told it was too risky as her movement and speech could become impaired. She revealed that she wanted to be cremated and where to sprinkle the ashes; she was an organ donor (her dad feels she had foreknowledge). On the morning of May 24, Kirsty's eldest daughter attempted to wake her. She couldn't! At the age of 35 Kirsty was dead. She was beautiful. A mother of three young children, in love with her husband, she had everything to live for.

Before the grief set in, all we wanted were answers. At first, we thought she may have died from an aneurism, heart attack, or maybe sleep apnea. The initial autopsy was inconclusive. We requested further testing. Her autopsy report indicated the likely cause was SUDEP. What in heaven's name was SUDEP? An urgent meeting with Kirsty's neurologist revealed that people do die unexpectedly from epilepsy, often during their sleep. Thank goodness we also learned Kirsty's condition was not hereditary but congenital. Her identical twin sister did not have it!

Grieving took on different dimensions for the family. Kirsty's twin was overwhelmed by sadness. Kirsty's younger sister sought the help of clairvoyants; she still wanted to communicate with her sister, much to the amusement of some and concern of others. Kirsty's husband threw himself into raising their three children aged 5, 7 and 9. Kirsty's dad couldn't talk about it. I devoured books on grieving and research on epilepsy. We all muddled along with support from family and friends.

Although the grieving is less, we continue to mourn our loss. Kirsty's twin is still angry that we weren't told about SUDEP. However, I'm not sure knowing would have changed things. I would have hated to see Kirsty being treated as a person with an illness – being watched.

My initial fears and sadness were that Kirsty would be forgotten, that she would not be there for her children and they would never know their mother. So I decided to compile Kirsty's Memoirs (contributions from friends and family). Publishing the Memoirs not only provided us all with a positive outlet for our grieving, it was also another way of capturing the wonderful memories. Kirsty is not forgotten!

Janine Mifsud

Seizure-related respiratory factors in SUDEP

Respiratory dysfunction during a seizure or in the immediate post-seizure period may contribute to SUDEP in a subset of patients with uncontrolled seizures. We have investigated the incidence and severity of seizure-related respiratory dysfunction in patients with medically refractory partial epilepsy admitted to the epilepsy monitoring unit (EMU) for characterization and localization of seizures as part of a presurgical evaluation.

In a large study, looking at over 300 seizures in 56 patients, we showed that blood oxygen saturation dropped below 90% in about one-third of seizures. These drops in oxygen saturation (hypoxemia) occurred whether or not the seizure progressed to a generalized convulsion. In a subset of these seizures, the hypoxemia was very severe (below 70%). Hypoxemia was more likely to occur in males, in temporal lobe onset seizures, in right hemisphere onset seizures and in seizures that spread from one hemisphere to the other. There was a cessation of breathing (central apnea) with most seizures that were accompanied by hypoxemia (Bateman, Li & Seyal et al. 2008).

We have shown that seizure-related hypoxemia is accompanied by a rise in carbon dioxide levels in expired air (hypercapnia). Again, in some seizures, this hypercapnia can be profound (exceeding 70 mm Hg). Marked abrupt rises in carbon dioxide are accompanied by severe changes in the pH of the blood (acidosis). The rise in carbon dioxide levels can last many minutes even though after the seizure both the depth and rate of breathing are enhanced relative to just before the seizure. This particular finding suggests that some seizures may result in persistent dysfunction of gas exchange mechanisms within the lungs (Bateman, Li & Seyal 2008, Seyal et al. 2010).

Most recently we have shown that there is an association between seizure-related hypoxemia and abnormalities in the electrocardiogram (EKG) during the recovery phase after a heart beat (repolarization abnormalities). In EKG recordings, repolarization abnormalities are demonstrated by measuring the QT interval. During seizures, we saw both a transient prolongation of the QT interval and a more persistent shortening of the QT interval, both of which were more likely to occur in seizures associated with hypoxemia (Seyal et al. 2011). It is known that abnormal prolongation of the QT and abnormal shortening of the QT increase the risk of significant cardiac arrhythmias that may result in sudden death (Schouten et al. 1991, Schimpf, Borggrefe & Wolpert 2008). Seizure-related hypoxemia and hypercapnia may thus increase the risk of potentially fatal cardiac arrhythmia.

In two cases of SUDEP recorded in two different EMUs, brain wave activity was suppressed following secondarily generalized convulsive seizures. Respiratory effort was present and EKG showed persistent cardiac activity for several minutes following the seizures. Oxygen saturation and carbon dioxide levels were not measured in these patients but EKG abnormalities suggesting effects of hypoxemia and acidosis on the heart muscle were present following both seizures (Bateman, Spitz & Seyal 2010).

Animal studies have suggested that a class of medications called selective serotonin reuptake inhibitors (SSRIs), commonly used to treat depression, may improve seizure-associated respiratory function (Tupal & Faingold 2006). In a retrospective study, we showed that patients taking SSRIs were less likely to have severe hypoxemia with partial onset seizures compared with patients not taking these medications. This protective effect was not evident in seizures that progressed to generalized convulsions (Bateman et al. 2010).

Our investigations suggest that seizure-associated respiratory dysfunction may have an important role in SUDEP in some patients. Large-scale studies with continuous monitoring of blood oxygen saturation, respiratory effort, and EKG in patients with uncontrolled seizures in the ambulatory setting are needed to better define the role of respiratory dysfunction in SUDEP.

Masud Seyal
Professor, Department of Neurology
University of California, Davis, USA.

Lisa M. Bateman
Assistant Professor, Department of Neurology
University of California, Davis, USA.

The role of serotonin in SUDEP

SUDEP is a diagnosis of exclusion (Nashef 1997). While a specific etiology for SUDEP has not been identified, it has been proposed that there may be cardiac (e.g. arrhythmias or arrest) or respiratory (e.g. respiratory arrest or hypoventilation) etiologies for SUDEP. Whether one of these is most important or each is equally important in causing SUDEP is yet to be determined. A primary cerebral etiology has also been proposed (e.g. 'electrical shutdown' of the brain or an arousal deficit), although this would only cause death if it led to cardiac or respiratory dysfunction. While the study of SUDEP is still in its early stages, several consistent risk factors have been identified through retrospective analysis of witnessed cases. These include sleeping face-down, being diagnosed with epilepsy at a younger age, having difficult to control seizures (i.e. requiring multiple antiepileptic drugs) and having generalized seizures (Tomson et al. 2008).

Since SUDEP is a diagnosis of exclusion and results in death, it does not lend itself well to designing controlled trials in patients. Therefore, developing animal models of SUDEP may prove useful. Several animal models have been shown to have seizure-related respiratory arrest that results in death if respiration is not supported. In one of these models, the DBA/2J model of sound-induced seizures, respiratory arrest can be prevented if mice are pretreated with the antidepressant fluoxetine, a serotonin selective reuptake inhibitor (SSRI) that increases the amount of the neurotransmitter serotonin available to act on neurons. In mice that did not have seizure-related respiratory arrest, it could be induced by pretreatment with a serotonin receptor blocker (Tupal & Faingold 2006). These results in mice are interesting, because many patients with epilepsy have apnea after seizures (Bateman, Li & Seyal 2008), and this apnea is reduced in patients taking SSRIs (Bateman et al. 2010).

That seizure-related respiratory arrest and death may be serotonin-dependent is intriguing, though not surprising. Serotonin is a well-known respiratory modulator, regulating breathing in order to maintain acid-base balance in the blood within a narrow range (Richerson 2004). Mice with genetic absence of serotonin neurons in the brain have a blunted respiratory response to inspired carbon dioxide (CO_2), an otherwise potent breathing modulator (Hodges et al. 2008). Serotonin is also a well-recognized modulator of cortical excitability which reduces susceptibility to seizures. In animal models, treatments that increase serotonin decrease seizure susceptibility. Conversely, decreasing serotonin function increases seizure susceptibility

(Bagdy et al. 2007). Interestingly, patients with epilepsy who take SSRIs, such as the aforementioned fluoxetine, tend to have improved seizure control (Kanner 2009).

Sudden infant death syndrome (SIDS) is another sudden death entity that is also a diagnosis of exclusion. Cardiac, respiratory and arousal/cortical activation etiologies have also been suggested for SIDS. Defects in the brainstem serotonin system are the most consistent finding in the brains of babies that die from SIDS. SIDS cases are also typically found face-down; a position that would lead to rebreathing of CO_2. Babies with an underlying defect in their brainstem serotonin system may not be able to detect the increased CO_2 resulting from rebreathing, so that they do not respond with an increase in breathing. Data from the genetically serotonin neuron deficient mice show that these neurons are also essential for waking up in response to increased CO_2 (Buchanan & Richerson 2010). Therefore these babies may not be able to arouse in response to the increased CO_2, so that they do not turn their head to relieve the cause of rebreathing. The defects in breathing and arousal together would cause them to become increasingly acidotic, and ultimately die from hypoxia (Kinney et al. 2009). Similar mechanisms could be at play in SUDEP (Richerson & Buchanan 2011).

It is likely that further studies in animal models, and validation in human patients, will lead to better definition of the mechanisms of SUDEP. This may then allow identification of those individuals at the highest risk of SUDEP in whom preventive measures can be implemented. Through this kind of research it is possible that this unnecessary cause of death might be eliminated.

Gordon F. Buchanan
Assistant Professor, Department of Neurology
Yale University, New Haven, CT, USA.

George B. Richerson
Professor and Head, Department of Neurology
Professor, Department of Molecular Physiology and Biophysics
The University of Iowa, Iowa City, IA, USA.

SUDEP and central nervous system function

In any death, there must be cessation of cardiac and respiratory function. In SUDEP, the mechanisms of failure of respiration and/or cardiac function during or after seizures, and what drive these, are unknown.

There is reasonable evidence now to suggest that there is cardiac and/or respiratory dysfunction during seizures and particularly during generalized tonic-clonic seizures, the seizure type that is most frequently associated with SUDEP. However, the high frequency with which cardio-respiratory dysfunction occurs is not reflected in SUDEP incidence figures which extrapolated to the population with refractory epilepsy, are still relatively low at 0.5-1/100 per year. Crucial additional seizure characteristics and epilepsy features that elevate peri-ictal cardio-respiratory dysfunction to critical, life-threatening proportions remain unidentified. SUDEP incidents witnessed in epilepsy monitoring units where recording of cardiac function (EKG) and brain function (EEG) suggest that in at least these SUDEP cases, the primary event is not cardiac. Unfortunately, definitive comment on respiration has not been possible in these comments as the essential parameters for doing so – oxygenation, respiratory rate/depth and end tidal CO_2 are not routinely recorded during seizure monitoring. However, the EEGs in many of these cases seem to point to profound post-ictal suppression of central nervous system function. Is this inordinate and especially pronounced in patients prone to SUDEP? Does the EEG provide an index for measuring risk? How does it relate mechanistically with the cardiac and/or respiratory dysfunction that constitutes the final common pathway? The answers have not been clear.

In one recent study of 10 definite SUDEP cases electro-clinical seizure features were studied to determine the role of EEG (Lhatoo et al. 2010). A generalized estimating equation (GEE) model was used to estimate odds of SUDEP using the duration of post-ictal EEG suppression (PGES) as a continuous and categorical variable. When only generalized motor seizures were studied, (cases = 16 seizures, controls = 58 seizures), PGES was found to be significantly longer in the seizures of cases than those of controls ($p < 0.001$). Durations of PGES >50 seconds had significantly elevated odds ratios (ORs). (OR = 5.25; 95% CI: 1.28–22.64; $p < 0.05$). OR increased exponentially with PGES >80 seconds (OR, = 19.29; 95% CI: 2.91–128.02). After adjustment for potential confounding variables, each 1-second increase in duration of PGES increased the odds of SUDEP by a factor of 1.7% (95% CI:1.005–1.027; p < 0.005) [25]. This study was retrospective and meaningful conclusions on the relationship of respiration to PGES cannot therefore be drawn but there is an urgent requirement for larger scale studies to confirm these findings. Unfortunately, the relatively low incidence figures in individual epilepsy practices mean that any such studies have to be carried out across many centres over several years, and in methodologically sound ways.

However, this preliminary study indicates that careful study of clinical features as well as peri-ictal EEG may yield clues to SUDEP pathogenesis and provide an individualized marker of SUDEP risk. The relationships between EEG suppression, brainstem function, central respiratory drive and cardiac function require careful study. The recently announced National Institutes of Health (NIH-USA) program for funding multi-centre, multi-disciplinary studies leading to the uncovering of SUDEP mechanisms and potential, evidence-based preventive measures in the future presents an opportunity for a comprehensive look at precisely these relationships.

Samden D. Lhatoo
Professor of Neurology
University Hospitals Case Medical Center, Cleveland, OH, USA.

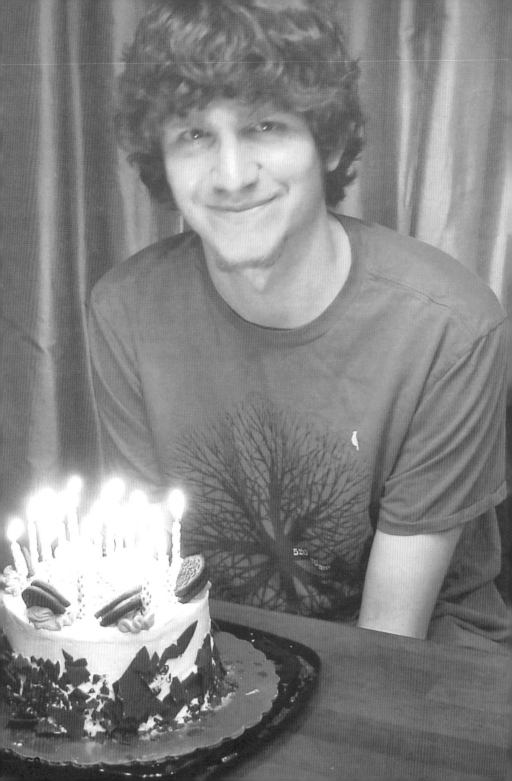

Tyler

Our son Tyler passed away on January 23rd 2011, from a seizure in his sleep, at the young age of 20. A sophomore at university, his death occurred on a Friday night and he lay in his bed face down for almost 48 hours in his college dorm room, alone. When residents thought something might be wrong, they called campus police and he was found. We had spoken to Tyler that Friday night via text messages. We wished him good night and told him that we loved him. No parent thinks about having to make funeral arrangements for their child.

Tyler had a febrile seizure at 19 months old. Ten years later he had his second seizure. Over the next seven years ambulance rides, emergency rooms, EEGs, MRIs, CT scans, hospital stays, and medication changes became the norm. The side effects from the medications, including memory and cognitive issues, were disheartening. A neurosurgeon pointed out a 'lesion' in Tyler's left temporal lobe and the discussion of surgery began. When we were told that after surgery 'he would never have seizures again', the decision was made for Tyler to have most of his left hippocampus removed. The recovery went well and we were hopeful, but three months later he had another seizure.

Tyler started College in 2009 and we constantly worried about him. He was having problems concentrating and remembering things for tests due to the meds. He especially enjoyed video games and in the future he wanted to write games. He became president of the Gamer's Club at school. One day Tyler passed out on the ice rink but no seizure was noted. The doctor recommended getting his heart checked but the tests were all normal. We were NEVER told that Tyler could die from epilepsy or a seizure. However, SUDEP is an acronym that we have come to know all too well in the days and months following his death

We are a devastated family and we are still in shock. It is just five months since his death. Holidays and his birthday which has just passed, bring bad days. A big piece of us was taken away. His room is untouched and we go in there and just sit. It smells like Tyler. The guilt, anger and the constant thoughts of what we should have done differently go through our minds every day. Tyler was patient, loving, gentle, and very smart. He had lots of potential. Now we visit the cemetery every weekend and take flowers.

We wish that we would have been told about SUDEP sooner. We would have done things differently. We have established a scholarship in Tyler's name at the University, for students with epilepsy. We want to keep Tyler's memory alive and show that he did not die in vain.

Mark and Coral Stevenson

61

SUDEP and nocturnal seizures

Individuals with epilepsy have a mortality rate 2-3 times that of the general population which can be attributed both to underlying disease but also to epilepsy itself. Sudden unexpected death in epilepsy (SUDEP) is the commonest category of seizure-related death.

A number of studies have identified frequent generalized tonic-clonic seizures as the most significant risk factor for SUDEP. The majority of SUDEP cases are unwitnessed and it has been noted that victims of SUDEP are often found in bed. In a study of SUDEP in a residential school for children with epilepsy who were closely supervised at night and carefully monitored following a seizure there was a lower incidence of SUDEP during term time and no witnessed deaths occurred raising the possibility that supervision and attention to recovery following a seizure and positioning or stimulation if necessary might play a role in SUDEP prevention (Nashef et al. 1995).

A large UK based case control study examining risk factors for SUDEP identified 154 cases from a variety of sources (Langan, Nashef & Sander 2005). The majority of victims (66%) were found dead in bed. Fifteen percent of deaths were witnessed and most of these occurred in association with a seizure. This study examined the potential role night time supervision might play in the prevention of SUDEP. Supervision at night, either by an individual in the same room or the use of special precautions such as a listening device was found to be protective.

Data from this UK case control study has recently been re-examined by Dr R. Lamberts and Dr R. D. Thijs from the Epilepsy Institute in the Netherlands Foundation with a view to determining whether victims of sleep-related SUDEP are more likely to have nocturnal seizures and whether there is a difference in seizure pattern, diurnal vs. nocturnal, between victims of SUDEP and controls who are living with epilepsy. This analysis has found that sleep-related cases of SUDEP were more likely to be unwitnessed and that such victims were more likely to have a history of nocturnal seizures. When other identified risk factors are controlled for, nocturnal seizures emerge as an independent risk factor for SUDEP. It was also noted that most sleep-related SUDEP cases occurred between 4am and 8am.

These findings reinforce the need for optimization of seizure control and raise again the somewhat thorny issue of night time supervision.

In addition it raises questions about the relationship between sleep and SUDEP and whether autonomic changes during sleep have a role to play in the genesis of SUDEP (Persson et al. 2007). A number of authors have commented on the fact that those with epilepsy may exhibit altered heart rate variability especially during sleep. Others have noted that SUDEP victims experienced a increase in heart rate during seizures that was higher with nocturnal seizures and that this difference in heart rates between nocturnal and daytime seizures was not identified in a control group of epilepsy patients. Further analysis of data from the UK case control study has identified that most sleep-related SUDEP deaths occurred in the early hours of the morning and this phenomenon has been noted in cases of sudden cardiac death and sudden infant death syndrome (Elliot 2001). Circadian patterns have not previously discussed in the context of SUDEP and this is an issue which warrants further examination.

Yvonne Langan
Department of Clinical Neurophysiology
St James's Hospital, Dublin 8, Republic of Ireland.

Can supervision prevent SUDEP?

There are at least two mechanisms of SUDEP: 1) brain activity affects heart activity both directly and via release of hormones that speed up the heart rate, leading to a dangerous change in heart rhythm which may occur during or after the clinical seizure, and 2) the respiratory centre in the brain stops working during a seizure and does not spontaneously recover.

Prevention of 1) could involve identification of those at risk by specialized tests and using medication to correct the abnormal heart rhythm. First aid might include staying with the person for a while after the seizure has apparently abated.

The second cause may explain why SUDEP is often unwitnessed. In some people seizure-related respiratory arrest is associated with EEG flatlining, with recovery occurring if the person is attended. Being rolled to the recovery position may be associated with breathing restarting and therefore may prevent this type of SUDEP, as the brain is stimulated by the passive muscle movement. Thus the issue of monitoring and accompaniment arises.

In our community-based epilepsy service in Cornwall UK we have only had one case of SUDEP in 14 years, although on epidemiological grounds we should have had 30-60 given the size of our clinical population and severity of their epilepsy. Our comprehensive approach to risk assessment and management can be summed up as follows:

■ *Optimize seizure control.* Seizure-related mortality can only happen if there are seizures. This is not just a responsibility for clinicians to ensure best possible treatment. People with epilepsy should know the reason for taking medication and understand the importance of seizure control. Failure to communicate this could lead to poor concordance and therefore increase the risk of death.

■ *People need to be able to make an informed choice about accompaniment and observation.* This requires a frank discussion about risks. Some clinicians seem to want to avoid having this discussion because of a fear of causing anxiety and of precipitating family tensions around the issue of overprotection. In practice I have not found this to be as difficult or as contentious as those who avoid having such discussion often seem to fear. Many people with epilepsy take the view that although the risk is real, it is nevertheless small, and outweighed by consideration of independence and quality of life, but these decisions are for the person with epilepsy to make, and not for the clinician to decide for them without discussion.

There are some monitoring devices that claim to detect seizure-like movement in bed or changes in breathing, heart rate or blood oxygen levels, in order to trigger an alarm. Some people find these useful but many find them intrusive. Problems arise both from false positive alarm activation and also where the alarm doesn't sound because sensitivity is reduced by specialized bedding. There is also a growing interest in seizure alert dogs and speculation as to whether they might reduce the risk of SUDEP, both by providing a warning of seizures and reducing seizure frequency. Robust clinical trial data is still lacking, and for the time being potential benefits must be regarded as theoretical rather than proven.

Although more information is needed regarding device sensitivity and effectiveness of seizure-alert dogs, decisions about deployment of these aids are for the patient; the clinician's role is to provide such information as is available. Some people with epilepsy may lack decision-making capacity due to intellectual disability or dementia, and many jurisdictions have a decision-making procedure allowing carers, clinicians, and other significant persons such as close relatives to act in the person's best interests (e.g. English Mental Capacity Act).

Professor Stephen Brown, Consultant Neuropsychologist (ret.)
Cornwall, UK.

Devices to detect apnea

Apnea occurs in SUDEP and, in some cases, is likely to be the primary event, with a cardiac arrest as a secondary event consequent to the cessation of breathing. It is well-known the cessation of breathing, apnea, occurs in many generalized and complex partial seizures, with associated lack of oxygen supply to the brain and heart. Apnea may result from airway obstruction, reduced respiratory drive or a combination of these. If recognized in time, however, death from apnea can be averted by prompt resuscitation.

Whilst monitoring of breathing is well-established in intensive care units, chronic monitoring in low intensity clinical, domiciliary and residential settings is not satisfactory. Existing devices that monitor respiration are based either on sensing airflow, movement, or concentrations of oxygen and carbon dioxide in the blood. The first approach uses detectors that are secured just under the patient's nose and sense the movement of air into and out of the airways to detect breathing. These can be successfully used within hospital, but difficulty keeping the device in place make it impractical for day to day use.

Other breathing detectors sense movements associated with breathing. They can be either attached to a mattress and with an audible or visible alarm triggered after a delay following cessation of movement; or a sensor pad on the chest which triggers when breathing is interrupted. The main problems with this approach are the false alarms that may occur, the size of the devices and need for mains power which restricts the places in which they may be used.

Pulse oximetry uses infrared light that shines through skin with good blood flow such as the finger, toe, or ear lobe, and can measure the oxygen level in the blood. The equipment is bulky, needs a mains power supply and the probes often get displaced from the skin.

There is an urgent need for a device that can reliably detect breathing and its absence, and which is small and discrete enough for long-term use in domestic and residential settings, as well as in low-intensity clinical care areas.

Electronic engineers at Imperial College and neurologists at UCL in London have pioneered a miniaturized, wearable apnea detection device and respiration monitor that is suitable for long-term use in low-intensity clinical, domiciliary or residential care and may alert carers to the cessation of breathing. The device is applied to the neck and detects the noise of respiration, is small and light enough to be worn comfortably and non-obtrusively, and is designed to reliably detect apnea, without false alarms. The device has just completed its first clinical trial at the National Hospital for Neurology and Neurosurgery, London in individuals with sleep apnea and will now be trialled in individuals with seizures that affect breathing. It is hoped that the device will be available for widespread use within two years.

John Duncan
Professor of Neurology
Deptartment of Clinical and Experimental Epilepsy
UCL Institute of Neurology, London, UK.

SUDEP and seizure prediction devices

Accurate prediction of seizures, and monitoring the occurrence of seizures in the ambulatory setting, has the potential to dramatically affect our understanding of the natural history of the condition, the relationship between seizure frequency, duration, memory and cognitive issues (Aldenkamp, Overweg & Gutter 1996), and perhaps into the phenomenon of SUDEP (Nilsson et al. 1999). Coupling such devices with other technologies may permit remote monitoring of cerebral and cardiac function through GPS and wireless communication systems, further improving patient safety. Given most episodes of SUDEP are unwitnessed, devices of this kind may shed light on the underlying pathophysiological processes involved.

Although the timing of seizures is generally regarded as unpredictable, there is evidence that changes occur in the brain's dynamical behaviour prior to attacks. Partly this evidence is provided by anecdotal reports of prodromes, featuring subtle changes in behaviour from sufferers and their carers in the hours or sometimes days before a seizure occurs. In addition, imaging studies have shown metabolic levels increase immediately prior to seizures (Zhao et al. 2007). Transcranial magnetic stimulation experiments have shown the brain is in a hyper-excitable state prior to seizures (Wright et al. 2006, Badawy et al. 2009). Other techniques, including functional magnetic resonance imaging, near infrared spectroscopy, auditory and visual steady-state responses, and direct electrical stimulation of the brain, indicate that cortical hyper-excitability is a precursor to epileptic seizures. This evidence suggests that seizures may be anticipated by tracking the excitability levels and dynamics of the brain. The reliable anticipation of seizures will allow patients to avoid dangerous situations, and potentially enable administration of a focal therapy, such as electrical stimulation or drug delivery.

The history of seizure prediction is chequered. Artifact and limited spatial resolution limit the utility of scalp EEG, and all current techniques use intracranial EEG data. The majority of previous approaches have typically used algorithms estimating entropy, correlation dimension, and short-term Lyapunov exponents (Babloyantz & Destexhe 1986, Pijn et al. 1991, Pritchard & Duke 1995, Casdagli et al. 1997, Le Van Quyen et al. 1999), and more recently interest has shifted to intracranial EEG synchronization analysis (Lai et al. 2003, McSharry, Smith & Tarassenko 2003, Winterhalder et al. 2003, Lai et al. 2004). Synchronization measures are thought to be correlates of cortical excitability reflecting the likelihood of seizure occurrence (Kalitzin et al. 2002). Although these algorithms have shown promise in certain patient groups, they have not delivered reproducible outcomes (Lehnertz et al. 2007, Mormann et al. 2003, Mormann et al. 2007). Although these methods are mathematically distinct, they are conceptually similar and focused on measuring the degree of order within the EEG, where a decrease in complexity indicates an abnormal hyper-synchronous state associated with a pre-seizure state.

Determining when seizures are going to occur may enable more informed pharmacotherapy to improve seizure control, possibly with fewer drug side effects. People with epilepsy may be able to make important changes to their activities and lifestyle in an appropriate time frame, based on the likelihood of seizure occurrence, for example avoiding swimming and retiring early when a high risk is indicated.

There is insufficient information as yet to comment definitively on the benefits of seizure prediction, but early studies with an implantable device are very positive (Davis et al. 2011). The algorithm assessment studies also provide strong evidence that the device will be effective as a seizure prediction system, which may lead to dramatically improved quality of life and reduce the risk of injury associated with unpredictable seizures. For many patients it is this intrinsic unpredictability that is the most disabling aspect of the condition (Rajna et al. 1997, Mormann et al. 2007, Schulze-Bonhage & Kuhn 2008). It may also provide new insights and potentially preventative strategies in SUDEP.

Mark Cook
Professor of Neurology
St. Vincent's Hospital, Melbourne, Australia.

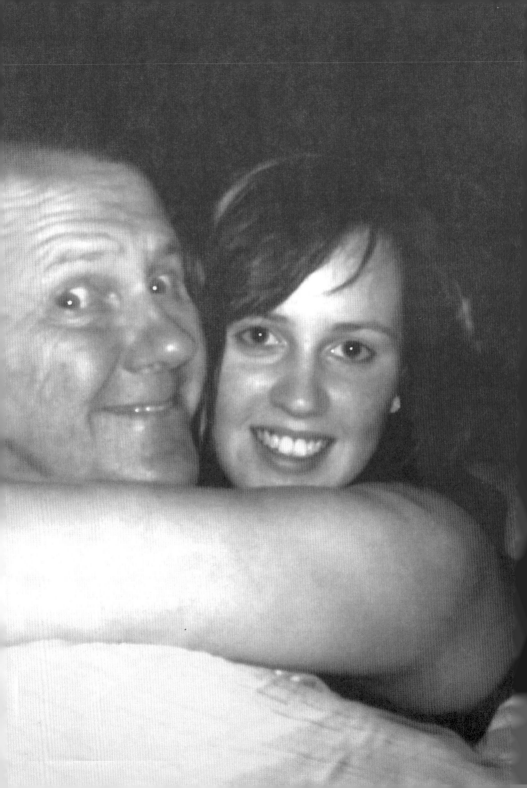

Jane

I am lying on her bed thinking of what we could have done to prevent her death. She was 19 years old. She had suffered from epilepsy since September 11, 2001; her first tonic- clonic seizure occurred while watching the Twin Towers fall to the ground. The doctors said it was not related to the terror in New York. They also told us 'you can't die from epilepsy'. Jane's seizures could be weeks, or months, apart. At times she had clusters (up to 4 per day) and recovery could take 3-4 days. She missed school and friendships suffered. Jane hated epilepsy, but she accepted it – to a degree.

The doctors tried different medications due to adverse effects like mood swings, depression and rashes. We thought the mood swings and depression were just normal teenage symptoms but I think the medications were more to blame than we realized or were told. At the time of her death Jane was taking three different medications. Unfortunately, the pills were a necessary evil.

Generally Jane's doctors were fantastic and I believe that the six or seven she saw over the years never considered SUDEP as a risk. Jane last saw a doctor about 6 weeks before her death and he thought that she may have been missing her medications but as far as we can tell she wasn't. I know this is often the case with SUDEP but we trusted her to self-medicate; after all she was 19 and already starting to organize her '21st'. Her doctors were as shocked by her death as we were.

There was no warning. The night before she died she went to dinner and the movies with her older sister, Laura. Meg, Jane's mother had been to an earlier session of the movie "Twilight" and she saw the girls in the queue going in. At midnight the girls arrived home and announced that they'd had an 'awesome' night. We chatted about the movie and went to bed.

The next morning Meg and Laura went off to work. I was on a day off and rose at about 9am. A friend arrived at 9.30am and I went to wake Jane for breakfast. She was dead!

The following months were a blur. The house was full of relatives and friends for a good 3 weeks. We have never seen so many flowers. The postie said he had never delivered so many cards to the one address. We had a private cremation with close friends and relatives, and later that day had a memorial service at a local church. I have never experienced a funeral like Jane's. Attended by some 450 people, Jane's school Principal and Deputy both spoke beautifully, the school choir sang hymns, family friends spoke, as did Laura, some cousins, and myself.

Jane would have been amazed that she had touched and affected so many and how they remembered her wonderful smile. Life's just not fair.

David McLachlan

71

Antiepileptic drugs, compliance and SUDEP

At least three categories of risk factors are operative in mechanisms for SUDEP (Lathers, Schraeder & Bungo 2008, 2011): arrhythmogenic (autonomic neural and cardiac function), respiratory and hypoxia, and psychological (stress, anxiety, depression). Arrhythmogenic risk includes subcategories: pharmacological drug effects, genetic ion channelopathies, and acquired heart disease.

The role of antiepileptic drugs (AEDs) in cause and/or prevention of SUDEP is not clear. Each patient, each AED, and combinations of AEDs need to be examined carefully to determine how best to individualize benefit/risk ratios. Individualized medical care minimizes the risk of unwanted AED side effects and seizure, thus preventing SUDEP. Such personalized care can be guided with therapeutic monitoring, indirectly addressing the unknown genetic role. The inter-individual variability in the pharmacokinetic properties and narrow therapeutic range of the older AEDs requires therapeutic monitoring to determine if serum levels will produce an optimal response in a given patient. With newer AEDs, monitoring is used to determine the individual reference concentrations based on intra-individual comparisons of drug serum concentrations. Therapeutic drug monitoring is used whether or not there is a well-defined therapeutic range. Since newer AEDs possess different pharmacological properties, the value of therapeutic monitoring must be assessed individually.

Drug therapies may increase or decrease SUDEP risk. The reputed advantage of newer drugs is less adverse events of sedation which may minimise noncompliance. Many new AEDs also have less frequent interactions, leading to improved tolerability with comedication (Lathers, Schraeder & Claycamp 2003, Walczak 2003). However, difficulty in achieving therapeutic dosage with some of the newer AEDs because of side effects makes one question whether some newer agents are 'better' than the older AEDs. Newer AEDs, such as topiramate and lamotrigine, developed for chronic focal and secondarily generalized epileptic seizures, do not seem to have a better therapeutic efficacy than traditional anticonvulsants such as phenobarbital.

Risk of SUDEP rates in patients on lamotrigine, gabapentin, topiramate, tigabine, zonisamide are similar to those on standard AEDs. This suggests SUDEP rates reflect population rates and is not a specific drug effect. The US Federal Drug Administration requires this information be provided on warning labels with each above mentioned drug (Lathers & Schraeder 2002).

Studies have shown that beta blockers exhibit anticonvulsant activity and may decrease the risk of SUDEP. Additionally, beta blockers reduce stress and persons with epilepsy generally are stressed (Lathers 2011). Should persons at risk for SUDEP be placed on a beta blocker in addition to the prescribed anticonvulsant(s)?

Compliance with AEDs is important to prevent SUDEP. A Coroner's Office review of forensic cases in Allegheny County for the year 2001 (Lathers, Schraeder & Claycamp 2003, Koehler et al. 2010), found low or no levels of AEDs post mortem in persons who died of SUDEP. Hughes (2009) deemed the most important SUDEP risk factor to be noncompliance with antiepileptic medication. Ryvlin, Tomson and Montavont (2009) found SUDEP risk increased in patients with poor compliance and nocturnal, generalized tonic-clonic seizures. Maintaining stable therapeutic drug levels is crucial to avoid SUDEP. Noncompliance with AED medication may be the most important (Hughes 2009) or one important risk factor for SUDEP (Lathers & Schraeder 2011b).

Compliance is not the only risk factor to be addressed if a person is a SUDEP victim. Clinical pharmacology questions to be asked post mortem (Lathers & Schraeder 2009) include: evaluation of AED dose; the actual AED or AED combinations used; possible drug-drug interactions; were the levels of AEDs below the lower level of quantification of the assay method post mortem; and whether there was a recent change in the AED dose or AEDs prescribed? When considering the role of drugs as protectors of life, clinical pharmacologists emphasize use of all drugs is a risk/benefit ratio evaluation and that AEDs may not provide 100% protection against sudden death. Prompt and optimal control of interictal and ictal epileptogenic activity will prevent SUDEP. AEDs and compliance or lack thereof, must be further evaluated as a major SUDEP risk factor.

A global focus must be the identification of risk factors for and mechanisms of sudden death in epilepsy (Lathers 2009).

Claire M. Lathers
Emeritus Fellow in Clinical Pharmacology
Albany, NY, USA.

Mortality and nonadherence to AEDs

Epilepsy is widely known to be associated with increased mortality and morbidity: A review of the epidemiological literature indicates that patients with epilepsy have a nearly threefold increase in mortality compared with the general population (Nei & Bagla 2007). There are many factors contributing to the higher risk of death in patients with epilepsy, but a lack of seizure control is a major one (Forsgren et al. 2005). Patients with uncontrolled seizures may also face a greater risk of physical injuries, such as fractures, falls, head trauma, motor vehicle accidents, occupational injuries, and burns, as well as various psychosocial morbidities including depression, anxiety, and social ostracism (Sperling 2004, Kwan & Brodie 2007). These injuries and morbidities often translate into increased utilization of emergency departments and inpatient services, as well as higher costs for insurers and other stakeholders in the health care system.

The effectiveness of antiepileptic drugs (AED) is limited if patients do not adhere to their regimens. The general estimates of epilepsy patients' adherence to medication regimens vary but tend to be less than optimal: In one patient survey, more than 70% of respondents reported they had omitted doses of their AEDs (Cramer, Glassman & Rienzi 2002). Other studies, using insurance-claims databases, have reported that approximately 30% to 50% of patients with epilepsy do not adhere to their medication regimens (Rosenfeld, Bramley & Meyer 2004, Davis, Candrilli & Edin 2007).

The relationship between medication adherence and mortality or morbidity has been examined in other disease areas, but it has not been well explored in the context of epilepsy. With Dr. Edward Faught, formerly the director of the Epilepsy Center at the University of Alabama, Birmingham, and now a professor of neurology at Emory University School of Medicine in Atlanta, Georgia, we undertook a series of studies with two objectives: the first was to investigate whether nonadherence to AEDs is associated with increased mortality; the second was to examine whether nonadherence increases the risk of serious clinical events such as emergency department visits, hospitalization, injuries from motor vehicle accidents, fractures, and head injuries.

In the RANSOM studies (Research on Antiepileptic Nonadherence and Selected Outcomes in Medicaid) (Faught et al. 2008, Faught et al. 2009), we analyzed claims data from three US state Medicaid programs: Florida, New Jersey, and Iowa. The data sets contained complete medical and pharmacy dispensing claims for eligible people from January 1997 through June 2006, and included more than nine million covered lives. The study population was selected based on the following criteria: at least 18 years of age; at least one neurologist visit with a diagnosis of epilepsy or nonfebrile convulsions; at least two pharmacy dispensings of selected antiepileptic drugs (following a diagnosis of epilepsy/seizure); and at least six months of continuous Medicaid enrollment before the first post-epilepsy/seizure AED dispensing.

Based on these criteria, a total of 33,658 patients were included in our study population. Data from each patient were partitioned into 90-day quarters, and for each quarter in which a patient received treatment, his or her adherence was calculated according to the number of days' supply of antiepileptic drugs. According to our findings, patients did not adhere to their prescribed AED regimens in 26% of the quarters. We observed a total of 5,405 deaths in the study population; 1,691 of those deaths occurred during AED adherent periods, 2,797 during nonadherent periods, and 917 during untreated periods. When we adjusted for age, gender, and other potential confounders, we found that AED nonadherence (independent of nonadherence to medications in general) was associated with a threefold increased risk of mortality relative to adherent behaviour. Nonadherent individuals in the study group also experienced a 50% higher incidence of emergency department visits, an 86% increase in hospital admissions, and more common occurrences of fractures and injuries from motor vehicle accidents compared with patients who did adhere to their drug therapies.

Earlier research shows that patients' nonadherence to AEDs is correlated with increased health care utilization, suggesting an association with negative clinical outcomes and increased medical costs (Davis, Candrilli & Edin 2007). Our findings support that connection: nonadherence was associated with various cost increases – inpatient costs per quarter rose more than $4,000, and emergency department service costs rose more than $300 per quarter. Meanwhile, we observed lower costs for outpatient and pharmacy services, likely because of the nonadherent behaviour.

In order to better protect patients, it is vital to understand what factors drive nonadherence, and for clinicians, funding bodies, and drug innovators to use this knowledge to promote treatment strategies for epilepsy that offer increased likelihood of adherence.

Mei Sheng Duh, Paul E. Greenberg, Annie Guerin and Caroline Korves
Analysis Group, Inc., Boston, MA, USA.

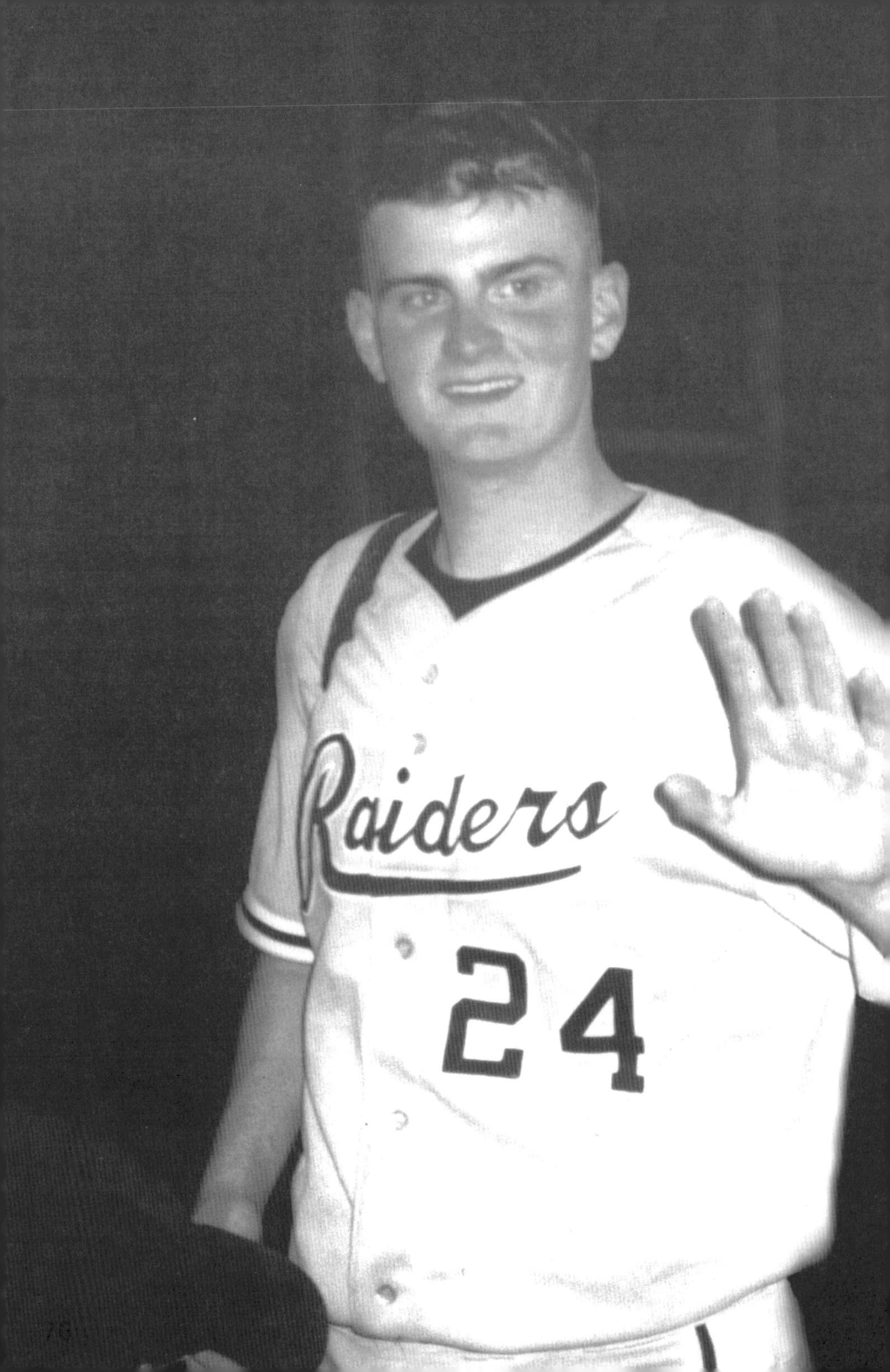
Raiders
24

Christopher

It was late in the afternoon on February 21, 2002 when the phone rang in my office. I picked up the receiver and my daughter, Lauren, was screaming, 'Jen just called and they can't get Christopher to breathe.' I had no idea who she was talking about. The moment our lives changed forever, suspended in time for that one brief second. And then I knew.

Christopher had been studying in bed and filling out an application for a summer internship. He was alone. His girlfriend found him. It was too late. He was dead. Autopsy results were consistent with SUDEP. We were stunned and confused. What was SUDEP? How could this have happened?

Christopher was 21 years old, a senior in college, facing a future of exciting challenges and endless possibilities. He approached life with passion and joy. He was competitive in the classroom. He loved playing baseball.

Christopher loved his family and friends. He had an opinion on everything, from politics to food to music to sports. Like others his age, he soaked up life and wanted it all.

And, Christopher had epilepsy. Diagnosed just before his senior year in high school, Christopher struggled with the side effects of his medication, the frustration of not being able to drive for extended periods, and the fear and uncertainty of when that next seizure would come.

Initially, Christopher's seizures were well controlled with medication but then he began to experience breakthroughs, and other medications were added. Finally, we believed we had the right combination, that he was seizure-free. However, after his death, we learned that the seizures had never stopped. They were coming more regularly, with greater intensity. The medication was not working. He did not share this information with his doctor or us.

Why? I can only imagine that he just wanted to live a normal life; that he felt he could figure it all out. He certainly never thought he could die from a seizure.

Would it have made a difference if Christopher knew about SUDEP? Would he have told us that his seizures were continuing? I believe he would have, but I'll never know.

There is nothing worse than losing a child but to feel that Christopher did not have all the information he needed to make informed decisions makes it especially cruel. He didn't have a level playing field. Knowing this information may have saved his life…what do you do with that?

Jeanne Donalty

The future of SUDEP research

Over a century since Spratling recognized that seizures can take a life suddenly and without warning, medical science has made limited progress. Modern epidemiological studies confirm Spratling's observations that tonic-clonic seizures are the most important risk for SUDEP and observational data from SUDEPs and near-SUDEPs confirm Spratling's principal antecedent of death is seizures (Spratling 1904).

Seizures, especially tonic-clonic seizures, can induce respiratory, cardiac and other autonomic changes, and shut-off the brain. These are prime candidate mechanisms for why some seizures are deadly. But some SUDEPs may not follow seizures (Donner, Smith & Snead 2001) and even video EEG recordings with physiological data fail to identify the mechanism of death. The need for progress grows as the magnitude of the problem is revealed, but the path for progress is unclear. Do we focus on collecting systematic SUDEP data, hoping for new insights? Do we study mouse models of early life epilepsy to understand why they die so young? Do we focus on ion channelopathies? Should we focus on seizures and respiration since this is where the data seem to be leading?

Epidemiologic and observational data suggest strategies to reduce SUDEP. Since seizures precede the vast majority of SUDEPs, preventing seizures, especially tonic-clonic seizures, may reduce risk. Better adherence with medication, a lifestyle that reduces seizure risk (e.g. sleep deprivation, stress, excess alcohol, etc), therapeutic approaches that better control refractory epilepsy (e.g. high dose or multi-antiepileptic drug regimens, epilepsy surgery), and monitoring of individuals with nocturnal seizures are all reasonable approaches, but there is no scientific evidence that any approach actually works. Future research should prospectively evaluate all such possibilities.

A significant practical problem in studying SUDEP mechanisms and prevention is that, thankfully, it is relatively infrequent. Therefore, testing interventions that hope to reduce SUDEP rates by half could require thousands of people to be followed for many years. This would obviously be expensive and time consuming. Consequently, SUDEP prevention studies are likely to be done in patients who are at very high risk (e.g. frequent tonic-clonic seizures) or on identified surrogate endpoints, (ictal or post-ictal physiological or biochemical changes that are most associated with high rates of SUDEP). However we need further research before we undertake even these modest studies. There is a need to:

- develop stronger international collaborations incorporating the expertise of cardiologists, pulmonologists, geneticists, biomedical engineers and others;

- obtain better prospective data from medical examiners, epilepsy centres, neurologists, community physicians, patients and families;

- perform prospective studies in epilepsy monitoring units using physiological parameters (e.g. video EEG, respiratory and cardiac data, sleep architecture, etc.) to improve our understanding of SUDEP mechanisms and identify surrogate physiological endpoints (e.g. specific cardiac, respiratory or EEG changes) for SUDEP to make intervention trials feasible;

- perform studies in epilepsy monitoring units to assess the effects of intervention during or after seizures to reduce physiological changes believed to increase SUDEP risk;

- study mechanisms and preventive strategies in relevant animal models;

- develop reliable devices to detect convulsive or nonconvulsive seizures;

- develop and study interventions to prevent the progression to SUDEP once a seizure has been detected; and

- facilitate better exchange of ideas between animal and clinical researchers.

Sadly, major advances in reducing SUDEP do not appear in the near future. Hopefully, this assessment is wrong. If not, we need to combine the passion of affected families with a vigorous effort by research teams. All researchers should hope for another team to discover a way to reduce SUDEP as soon as possible, but do everything ethical science allows to get there first. Collaboration, competition, sustained focus, and funding are a potent formula. Major advances in medicine sometimes come from systematic study with steady accumulation of data but sometimes big discoveries come from the periphery of the mainstream. We need to hedge our bets and support both front-runners and carefully choose long-shots.

Orrin Devinsky
Professor of Neurology, Neurosurgery & Psychiatry
NYU Langone School of Medicine, NY, USA.

Daniel Friedman
Assistant Professor of Neurology
NYU Langone School of Medicine, NY, USA.

Part 3.

facing the future

SUDEP: out of the shadows

In 1996 an international SUDEP workshop was held in London. Discussion included the urgent need for: a clear definition; an expansion of research; and the development of accurate, accessible SUDEP information. At that time SUDEP was rarely mentioned on any website, but in 2011 it can be found on websites worldwide. Unfortunately the accuracy of the material varies.

The UK has led the way in producing quality SUDEP information for the public and health professionals, raising public awareness, supporting the bereaved, and instigating strategic action at a policy level. The work of Epilepsy Bereaved has been recognized with an award from the Queen and organizations in Ireland, Australia, Canada, the USA and elsewhere have taken their lead from the UK movement. Cooperation between the UK and Australia led to the publication of the first 'global conversation' book in 2005, and in 2011 this collaboration has extended to include Canada in the production of a second book. This new publication has a vital role to play in explaining the research evidence to general audiences, including people affected by epilepsy and health professionals.

Despite this improved community awareness the need for individualized communication about SUDEP remains essential for people with epilepsy. Warnings from some that doctors could be sued if they talked to patients has never been supported by any jurisprudential precedent and thankfully this argument has now disappeared from clinical reviews. The focus now is on how to communicate risk in line with the scientific advances on risk factors of SUDEP (Hanna & Panelli 2010). Reducing the number of seizures is certainly the most likely way of reducing deaths until more evidence emerges (Doheny 2011). Whilst epilepsy surgery may be an option for some people at `high risk', simple measures may include attention to self-management behaviours of the larger population of people `at risk'.

A USA workshop in 2008 involving clinicians, epilepsy organizations, patients and families concluded that some of the benefits of communication about SUDEP included patients sharing the treatment goals with the physician and increased opportunity for patients to make informed decisions on self-management and adherence.

Openness about SUDEP requires information to be provided and available as part of routine epilepsy information. Research from risk management across other health conditions supports a multi-disciplinary approach. The team member responsible for communication may vary in each setting but, left unplanned, there is a risk that the conversation never takes place. Some clinicians use patient-led counselling check lists including SUDEP. Others encourage discussion of epilepsy-related fears including loss of predictability and death. Anxiety about fatality is common across many health conditions, but research shows that it can be temporary and part of natural adaptation to illness. Patients can benefit from the opportunity for frank discussion. Experts in risk communication advise that success requires an agreed basic core of information which identifies the nature and severity of the potential harm. Epilepsy mortality is well recognized in the scientific literature as a severe harm. The information needs to include the likelihood of harm under various circumstances and the possibility and difficulty of reducing that harm. Odds and percentages are not generally understood.

There are situations where, a clinical decision may be made that there is a good reason why information should be withheld or communication should be deferred. This point was explored at the USA SUDEP workshop and it was recognized that exceptions would include individual patients with unique psychosocial or cultural contextual features.

In consideration of bereaved families, Epilepsy Bereaved supports national guidelines in England and Wales that include signposting to SUDEP support services. This recognizes the trauma and complexity of grief that is associated with a SUDEP death. Families experiencing SUDEP report a lack of SUDEP knowledge in their communities including, on occasion, in criminal inquires. They need help to understand what has happened and support during investigation of the death and their journey of bereavement. Many are helped by meeting others who have experienced SUDEP and consoled by the opportunity to contribute to research and influence change.

SUDEP is finally coming out of the shadows, but this is just the beginning. SUDEP awareness must now lead us on to a reduction of epilepsy-related deaths and enhanced quality of life for people living with epilepsy

Jane Hanna
Epilepsy Bereaved

SUDEP: going public

The general community does not fully appreciate the nature of epilepsy, or its impact including the risk of epilepsy-related death. This lack of understanding is reflected in inadequate health policies, inaccurate or biased media reports and the disbelief of others when a family bereaved by epilepsy attempts to explain an epilepsy-related death.

Altering community perceptions is a challenge.

Should you try to mount a major awareness campaign aimed at the entire community or do you target specific groups? If you focus on the community as a whole, it can be difficult to communicate complex messages and there will be individuals in the community for whom the general message triggers a need for more individualized information. In practice, it is essential to run several layers of information at the same time. While putting our some very general messages to the public at large, it is necessary to have prepared stakeholders, including health professionals to handle public and patient inquiries. Following the UK audit of epilepsy-related deaths, Epilepsy Bereaved ensured that alongside the public campaign to publicise the results, all epilepsy organizations agreed on key messages. A helpline was established with staff trained to handle any public response generated by the larger campaign, and it functioned very effectively.

National media reporting of SUDEP is easiest to achieve in the early years of a public education campaign. In the UK, Epilepsy Bereaved continues to attract about 7 national media stories a year (with a circulation of about 5 million) but success depends on something new to report. Local reporting of SUDEP is easier to achieve and may be most effective in meeting the aims of public education. A SUDEP death often has a deep impact on a local community. This can evoke a desire to understand the circumstances and to provide support for those affected.

Targeting of specific audiences is important in influencing professionals, opinion leaders or policy makers with power to elicit change. Those targeted in the UK have included the voluntary sector, government, coroners, pathologists and health professionals. Key messages, although adapted for each audience, have included the impact of SUDEP, risk reduction strategies and the urgent need for further research and monitoring.

At the national level, Epilepsy Bereaved convenes Parliamentary receptions and provides evidence on epilepsy mortality to the Epilepsy All Party Parliamentary Group, most recently presenting a 2011 national mortality statement signed by the President of the British ILAE, SUDEP researchers, clinicians, and politicians.

Local government campaigns are of increasing importance in England as health care reforms decentralise power. Variations in deaths statistics between local health providers, and high costs of unplanned Accident and Emergency services in many regions, may influence health managers to redesign services which will be able to support identification and stepping up of care for people with epilepsy in the community who are at risk.

Positive outcomes in the UK which have resulted from the national audit and subsequent Epilepsy Bereaved campaigns include: national guidelines recognizing SUDEP as essential information; the prioritization of SUDEP Awareness in epilepsy campaigns by the Joint Epilepsy Council; risk reduction and SUDEP as part of epilepsy service planning in Wales; pathology guidelines on investigation and reporting of epilepsy deaths; and increased coronial reporting to UK health regulators.

In any SUDEP campaign, the bereaved can be powerful advocates on behalf of people with epilepsy. In the UK, families who are willing and considered ready to share their stories are supported to participate. They have been successful in engaging politicians and the media and some go on to become volunteer regional ambassadors.

In future, the explosion of internet sites, and social networking, is likely to be an increasingly powerful influence on public perceptions. The 'global conversation' book, and its ongoing website will have a vital role in continuing the promotion of responsible and accurate public information on SUDEP.

Fiona McDonald
Communications Manager
Epilepsy Bereaved, UK.

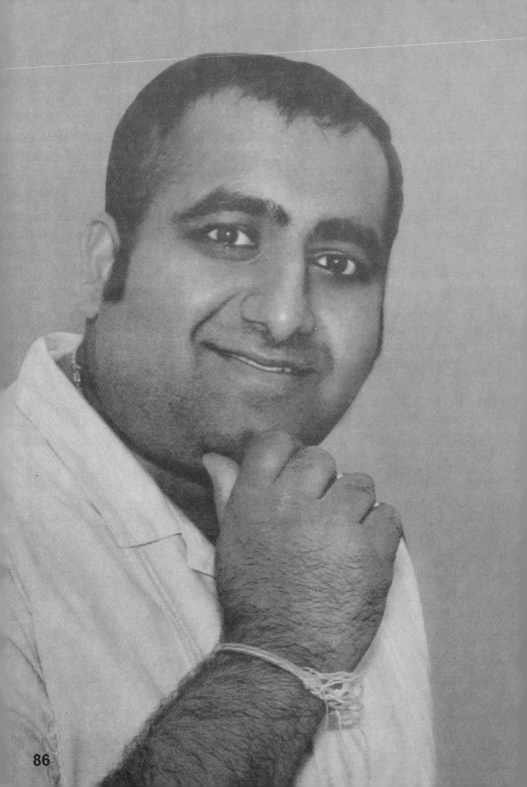

Ravin

On the 12th February 2011 at approximately 6:00pm, our brother Ravin J Dattani sadly passed away. He was 29 years old. The exact cause of death is unknown as of yet; however the signs point to SUDEP. Ravin's epilepsy started when he was 15 years old; he accepted it, and never let it rule his life.

Ravin was one of twelve grandchildren. The most important people in his life were his wife Reshma, dad Jayanti, mum Kirti, and younger sister Jalpa, along with his extended family.

Ravin's instinct was to protect and look after people. This was due to his upbringing and the values his parents instilled in him from a young age. Ravin and Jalpa shared a deep bond, they would not need to show it, but you could tell instantly how much Ravin loved Jalpa and how he always wanted to be there for her and protect her.

Ravin was the rock of the family. He took each and every family member under his wing, comforting, supporting, and directing us, no matter what.

Though we are all cousins, we are as close as brothers and sisters. One of the main reasons why we see ourselves in that way is due to Ravin. He always made sure we knew that family is the most important thing in the world, and in this respect it made us want to be more like him. For that Ravin, we thank you.

In all aspects of life Ravin showed strength of character, determination and always displayed perseverance in the face of adversity. Ravin never let it show when he was feeling down. He would bring warmth into the room with his gentle smile and heart of gold. We want to thank you Ravin, for being our brother, our friend, our teacher, and our sunshine when it was raining.

The family has been supported by Epilepsy Bereaved, and we believe the work they do in raising awareness about SUDEP and in providing support for families, is invaluable.

Ravin's loss is felt by so many; we want other families to be aware of SUDEP. Thirty six of us, including family, extended family and friends, came together in July 2011 to participate in the British London 10k run, and we will continue to raise money and awareness in the future, in order to help others who have been bereaved through epilepsy.

Life has changed, everything has changed. We are the people we are today, due to the great influence Ravin had in our lives.

The Dattani Family

SUDEP: a clinician's perspective

Although SUDEP had been recognized and quantified in the UK for some time, as recently as the mid 1990's no one in the UK was routinely discussing the concept or its implications with patients. The last two decades have seen health services introduce a number of guidelines across the UK. For doctors in Scotland, the first and leading one was produced by the Scottish Intercollegiate Guideline Network (SIGN 2003). As part of guideline number 70 (SIGN 70 – Diagnosis and Management of Adults with Epilepsy www.sign.ac.uk) a list was compiled of subjects that should be discussed with patients with newly diagnosed epilepsy.

This late acceptance of the importance of SUDEP discussions is a result of synergy between various parts/sections/collaborations within the voluntary sector. The 2003 SIGN guideline was compiled at about the same time as a verdict was produced from a high-profile inquest into the death of a patient with epilepsy. The ongoing focus on SUDEP helped cement its place in the list of information that should be offered in the time following a new diagnosis of epilepsy. The voluntary sector has played a key role in promoting the discussions; in addition to the mainstream epilepsy patient organizations, there has been prominent input from Epilepsy Bereaved UK, whose work has increased awareness of SUDEP among health professionals, policy makers and the community.

Clinicians will always have concerns about being forced to practice 'tick box' medicine, many with some justification. While guidelines have a role in contemporary medicine, everyone should remember that a guideline is a guide, an aid, a set of prompts, and not a list of mandatory instructions. While a frank discussion of the facts surrounding SUDEP may be best for many patients, some patients may not benefit from such an approach. For some, a diagnosis of epilepsy (or the experience of a single seizure) can be a psychologically fraught time, particularly following discussion of the many restrictions and cautions in lifestyle and career. Where the patient may be already overladen with doom, undue focus on the possible hazards could enhance the risk of negative effects such as depression, suicide attempts or reducing clinic attendance. For patients with no risk factors for refractory or particularly hazardous seizures, it may be more appropriate to focus on the likelihood of good drug response, and the positive steps that can be taken to promote and preserve optimal quality of life.

Intermittent high profile legal inquiries have continued to shape public opinion, leading to media coverage of death by seizure. Such stories may make good newspaper copy but do not always educate patients appropriately. The negative aspect is that such stories may mislead patients into thinking that they reinforce the notion of being in immediate peril.

The positive side effect is that media pressure impacts on government and policy-makers, leading to recognition in our National Health Service of the need for coherent and expert clinical response to epilepsy and first seizures. This has helped ensure that epilepsy care has improved across many regions of the UK in the last 20 years.

It is not appropriate for patients to obtain information about their possible epilepsy outcomes primarily through the media. Such issues deserve a measured discussion with their physician. An important part of the diagnostic visit is to uncover any latent morbid anxieties from both patients and their relatives. Management of such anxieties requires that the risks of seizures are properly contextualized, and where possible individualized. For some this will entail starker warnings than others – particularly where some aspects of behaviour or lifestyle will impact on seizure frequency or seizure severity. This will allow the potential for harm to be openly discussed – giving patients and relatives empowerment in its reduction.

Working in such partnership is one of the things that can make epilepsy clinics so rewarding for patient and doctor alike.

John-Paul Leach
Consultant Neurologist
Southern General Hospital and Western Infirmary, Glasgow, Scotland.

SUDEP: a general practice perspective

My interest in patients with epilepsy stemmed from an epilepsy audit in two general practices of 22,500 patients (Redhead et al. 1996) that demonstrated poor documentation and potential for improvement in care. Following this, a practice-based epilepsy clinic run by our epilepsy nurse specialist was established.

At a UK International League Against Epilepsy General Practitioner (GP) chapter meeting in 2010 I listened to a presentation from volunteers from Epilepsy Bereaved. A father, who had lost his teenage daughter asked 'Why did the doctors not tell us about the possibility of SUDEP?' He felt let down and betrayed. The implication was that doctors had a therapeutic privilege and had decided not to share it. A presentation from a young man with epilepsy followed. His own brother had died from epilepsy. He explained that he had only become interested in learning about his condition when it was brought home to him that a seizure could be fatal.

SUDEP is sudden unexpected death in patients with epilepsy. There is uncertainty and unpredictability about the causes but suggested risks factors include; young adulthood, presence of convulsive attacks, poor seizure control, poor adherence, male gender, more than one antiepileptic drug, frequent dose change, alcohol abuse and learning difficulty (Walczak et al. 2001, Hughes 2009, Nilsson et al. 1999). Most deaths seem to occur in bed.

The UK National Sentinel Clinical Audit of epilepsy-related deaths estimated 1000 epilepsy deaths annually of which 500 are from SUDEP (Hanna et al. 2002).

I reflected with some guilt that I had not routinely discussed SUDEP with my patients. Why was this? In truth there is a lack of awareness of the incidence of SUDEP in primary care. It was more common than I had thought. Should I tell everyone with the disease and how should the subject be broached? Can I assume that this would have already been discussed with the specialist at the time of diagnosis or during follow up? Anyway, when would be the right time?

The purpose of discussing SUDEP is to reduce the risk by helping the patient to understand more about their condition. It is uncomfortable for a GP to break the news about a condition where he feels he has limited knowledge and fears upsetting his patient and their family. However the evidence is that the majority of patients with epilepsy are already afraid that they could die with their next seizure and are concerned that they could sustain brain damage (Mittan 1986). A question such as 'What are your concerns about epilepsy or having a seizure?' may be followed by 'loss of my driving license' but it may also reveal fear of 'dying from a fit'. Another way of introducing the subject may be to use a question such as 'Do you know about any serious effects of epilepsy which can occur rarely?' 'I would like to discuss these with you at some point would you like me to talk about them today?'

These sorts of questions will gather the ideas and concerns of the patient. In response, at the right time for the patient, the doctor or epilepsy nurse can provide information and support. The resources available from organizations within the voluntary sector can be signposted. Patients do have right to know this important information but it clearly needs to be handled sensitively with thought and planning. It is possible that in time there will be a medico-legal obligation to document discussion about SUDEP. The roles of primary and secondary care need to be clearly defined and GP commissioning may help plan pathways. However, whenever SUDEP is first discussed it should not be a 'tick box exercise' where the potential bombshell is thrown to the patient and family. Put over constructively and positively, a discussion about SUDEP can be used to inspire adherence and avoidance of risk factors.

Keith Redhead
General Practitioner
Kings Lynn, Norfolk, UK.

SUDEP: a personal perspective

Six years ago I had a complex partial seizure, which evolved into a secondarily generalized tonic-clonic seizure (GTC). The seizure had been caused by a meningioma in the right frontal lobe which was surgically removed one week later. I decided to take advantage of my post-operative recovery free time to catch-up with post-due manuscripts. One manuscript touched upon the topic of sudden unexpected death in epilepsy (SUDEP) for which I had to check some statistical data on its prevalence. As soon as I read the first paragraph, I experienced a feeling of panic which caused me to close the book immediately… It took me six weeks to be able to look at that data again.

I am an epileptologist and almost all the patients I treat suffer from epilepsy. I am well versed on the complications of epileptic seizures, including SUDEP and its literature, which I have discussed uncountable times (every time I see a new patient)… So what caused my reaction when I tried to review epidemiologic data of this complication of epilepsy? Was it my first realization that I was at an increased risk of dying after having had an epileptic seizure?

When I thought of the way my patients react when I bring up the issue of SUDEP (and I always do in the first or second visit), I could not remember a single patient appearing anxious or in a panic (I cannot exclude the possibility that at least some patients kept their fears and worries to themselves). On the other hand, having a discussion of 'the loss of predictability' of one's life has been in my experience the most predictable trigger of tears and strong emotional reactions in my patients. Clearly, the fears associated with SUDEP are part of the broader fears that encompass the loss of predictability. In fact, when I tried to understand my reaction to reading data on SUDEP that were not new to me, I realized that it was not the fear of dying which triggered my panicky reaction. Rather, it was the fact that the epileptic seizure I had three weeks before was forcing me to come to terms with 'unpredictability' from now on.

Thus, should clinicians discuss SUDEP with their patients and, if yes, when? There is no question that SUDEP is a complication of epilepsy that patients and their family must know about. Furthermore, in the era of the internet, it is only a matter of time for patients and/or their families to come across it, if not in a newspaper article like the one published a few months ago in *The New York Times*. Clearly, patients are more likely to deal better with their fears of death associated with their epilepsy from a careful explanation provided by their own physician than from reading about SUDEP in the internet or on a magazine.

Discussion of SUDEP must be incorporated in the patient's education of the consequences of having epileptic seizures. But such education must include preparing patients to accept the 'loss of predictability', as this is a pivotal step towards dealing with the diagnosis of epilepsy. And the acceptance of the 'loss of predictability' will help patients come to terms with SUDEP.

Andres M. Kanner
Professor of Neurological Sciences and Psychiatry,
Rush University Medical Center, Chicago, IL, USA.

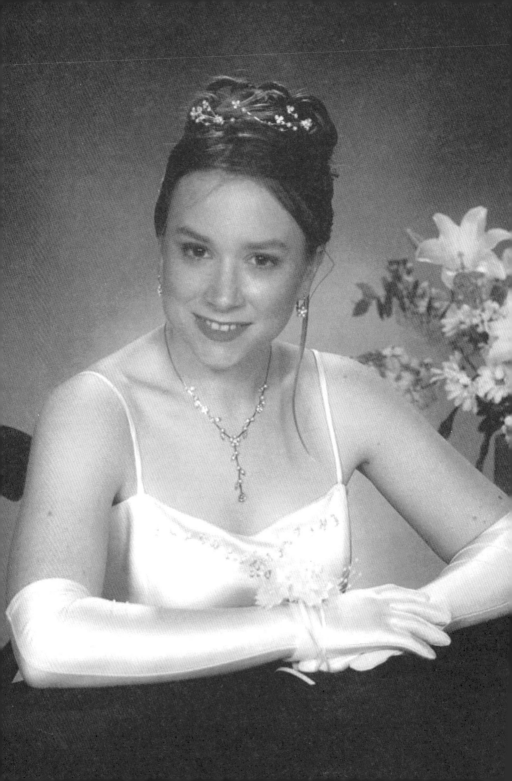

Kate

January 16, 2006 is the day that changed our family forever. It was the day we lost our vibrant, caring and precious, nineteen year old, only daughter Kate, and the loving sister of our three sons. We had only just left home, taking our seventeen year old son to the town hall for a presentation for his upcoming exchange year in Denmark, when we received a frantic phone call from our fifteen year old son, saying he couldn't wake Kate, even though the alarm kept ringing for her to get up to go to work. A week later, instead of farewelling our son for an exciting year away we were farewelling our beautiful daughter for ever.

She had been diagnosed at the age of six with epilepsy that mainly affected her in the REM stages of sleep. We were told she would grow out of it, and she did by the age of twelve. However, at sixteen it was to return in an adult form, again mainly affecting her when she had gone to bed. Sometimes she was aware that a seizure was about to happen and would get up to tell us, but once she slipped behind the door and we couldn't reach her. For safety reasons, she began to taking a mild anti-seizure medication twelve months prior to her dying and this had easily become part of her regular daily routine. She only had seizures when she was particularly tired and especially if the weather had been hot.

Epilepsy never stopped Kate living life to the fullest, studying nursing, working part-time at Subway and enjoying her family and many friends. She was so very comfortable with who she was and having epilepsy was part of that. She even counselled a young co-worker who had been diagnosed with epilepsy.

So why? No one ever told us that she could die from this, nor had we even heard of SUDEP till after her death. I often ponder, should we have known this, would we have allowed her to experience all those childhood joys of sleepovers and school camps? Would we tell another family with a child who had epilepsy? Of course we would.

We miss so much the joy and laughter she brought us, as her parents, her brothers and the many friends she had made. We only hope in telling Kate's story, awareness will be raised and other families spared the grief and heartache our family has endured.

Geoff and Wendy Leigh

SUDEP: risk perception and communication

Some physicians advocate talking about SUDEP risk with most (or all) patients with epilepsy and/or their caregivers. They argue that informed decision-making is otherwise impossible, or that the knowledge may lead to improved medication compliance and other behaviours that might reduce the risk of seizures and SUDEP. Other physicians believe the discussion is often unwarranted. They argue that the information can be emotionally damaging, or lead to overprotective behaviours, or that the information won't change behaviours and outcomes. Many physicians have questions about whether, when, and how to talk about SUDEP.

Behavioral decision theory can lend insight to this debate about risk perceptions, risk communication, and patient behaviour (Fischhoff 1999). Behavioral decision theorists assume peoples' actions are influenced by their 'mental models', the sets of beliefs intuitively drawn upon when deciding and behaving (Johnson-Laird 1983). When deciding what to do in a situation, our mental models include beliefs about our goals and available options, about the possible consequences of those options, perceptions of risk, and beliefs about causality (Morgan et al. 2002). Mental models evolve over time, changing with personal or observed experience, communication with others, and other forms of communication. Beliefs can also be influenced by emotions.

In new situations, people need to draw upon existing mental models that seem relevant. For example, new epileptic patients might apply existing mental models of medication in general to AEDs specifically. Some might believe, perhaps based on experience with other medicines, that there is no real harm in missing a dose (or several doses). If they miss a dose and do not have a seizure, such an erroneous belief may be reinforced.

Important gaps or misperceptions in mental models can lead people to make poor decisions, or to not even know that there are decisions to be made. For example, people can't choose to take precautions against a risk of which they are unaware. For a known risk, they can make a choice about using a preventive medication, technology or practice – but only if they know of it and have the information needed to judge its value. How effectively they use it depends on understanding when and how to do so. All of these decisions depend on their mental models.

While much remains unknown, evidence suggests that some behaviours such as consistent use of AEDs, night time monitoring, and assistance during seizures may reduce SUDEP risk. Families of some SUDEP victims report that they were never aware of the risk. Or, if they were aware, feel they did not sufficiently understand how to reduce it. They believe that they or their deceased loved-ones would have behaved differently, had their mental models not had critical gaps or misperceptions.

People want to make health-related decisions and engage in behaviours that help them reach their goals. Physicians play a crucial role in equipping patients with epilepsy to do that, via communications that address important gaps or misperceptions in their mental models. But first, the physician must know what those gaps and misperceptions are. A good starting point is to ask questions to elicit the patient's beliefs. Relevant questions to start with, and to return to periodically, might be: What do you think can happen if you have a seizure? How important is it to prevent seizures, and why? Can you do anything to prevent seizures? Do you think it matters if you miss a dose of your medication? Why?

Responses to such questions can allow physicians to assess and address important gaps and misperceptions in a specific patient's beliefs. Research on decision-making and behaviour suggests that this can help patients to make better decisions for themselves.

Laurel Austin
Assistant Professor
Copenhagen Business School, Denmark.

SUDEP: talking with adolescents

Being an adolescent with epilepsy carries a wide range of challenges for the young person with epilepsy, for the parents, and the health care professionals. Should we tell people with epilepsy that a considerable risk exists in regard to epilepsy or shouldn't we say? This question has baffled both parents and health care professionals for many years. Epilepsy is a highly individual diagnosis that carries different consequences from patient to patient. We could therefore argue that the information should also differ greatly.

Some see the large variation in the diagnoses as a reason to simplify the amount of information given by the health care professionals to adolescents with epilepsy. We feel that this is the wrong way to go about it. Today you can find an enormous amount of information regarding any subject on the internet and it is likely the most important tool young people use to find answers to their questions. It is however a setting where they are usually alone, and therefore not able to talk to others about some of the things they read.

It is important to plan how you inform the adolescent patient about the risks in epilepsy. In Norway we talk to teenagers about the risks in epilepsy in courses, in written material, on summer camps and in other arenas. Our experience is that young people are open to this information and able to understand the significance in the message about general risks and especially about SUDEP.

Much of the research on SUDEP tells us that seizure-freedom is important to reduce the risk for SUDEP. We also know that adolescents have a high rate of non-compliance. Many of the youngsters in Norway say that they would be more careful in taking their medications if they were adequately informed about the risks in epilepsy.

Working to empower young people with epilepsy is important to decrease the negative consequences of the social aspects of epilepsy. We know that epilepsy is associated with other negative factors such as unemployment, poor social skills and poor quality of life. Helping people with epilepsy to cope with the diagnosis and take control of their own lives must be one of our superior goals. By taking adolescents seriously and informing them about the different aspects of the epilepsy diagnosis, including the risks, we also empower young people to cope with the diagnosis in a better way.

Whilst we argue for the fact that young people need to be informed about the different aspects of epilepsy including the risks, we also feel strongly that it should not be done randomly. Talking about SUDEP is preferably done in a safe environment, in a small group with one or more health care professionals who have adequate knowledge on the subject, and who are experienced in talking to young people about difficult matters. There needs to be enough time set aside to give adolescents time to ask their questions, and preferably a follow-up session where subsequent questions may be asked. This type of meeting could, for instance, be arranged in cooperation with a patient organization and health care professionals.

Knowledge makes us stronger. Informing adolescents about the risks in epilepsy is important to give them a chance to make informed decisions about their life, and to empower them to become independent despite a diagnosis of epilepsy.

Stine Jakobsson Strømsø
Secretary General
Norwegian Epilepsy Association.

SUDEP: talking to patients and families

The discussion of potential death related to seizures must be presented with the greatest sensitivity based upon the likelihood of such a tragedy tempered by the physician's knowledge of the individual patient's/family's intellectual, psychological, and cultural needs.

Questions relating to this communication have been extensively discussed in a workshop dedicated to SUDEP (Hirsch 2011). Naturally, if a patient/family asks directly about the possibility of death related to seizures, the care provider is obligated to provide that information. When the question is not asked, should the issue be raised at all? This question was considered within the context of modern ethical thought regarding the right of the patient to know as well as the right not to know. The consensus opinion, although not unanimous, was that the reality of SUDEP should be discussed as it stresses to the patient the importance of seizure control, establishes a truth-telling relationship, provides an opportunity for the patient/family to express their concerns and potentially reduces the family's feeling of grief and blame should the event occur. The reasons to not offer this information centre on the possibility of introducing life-altering anxiety when the likelihood of SUDEP could be extremely low. Another reason offered is that, in certain cultures, discussing a possible event could be conceived as wishing or predisposing that event to occur. A major consideration that has been raised is that of 'the not asked question'. This refers to a patient/family having a fear about possible death, but being too afraid to ask about it. It has been the anecdotal experience of clinicians that the patient/family is actually relieved when the physician raises SUDEP, if only to express the very low risk of it occurring in appropriate situations.

The issue of when and how to discuss SUDEP is related, in part, to the degree of risk. It is generally agreed that discussion of SUDEP should occur as part of the education plan for all individuals with epilepsy. Such issues as first aid, adverse effects of antiepileptic drugs, driving and pregnancy, are frequently introduced during the first office visit, supplemented with written and other materials and then considered again during subsequent office visits. However, if the individual has tonic-clonic seizures which have been refractory to multiple medications, SUDEP should be discussed sooner rather than later. The discussion is of lower priority for the child with typical absence epilepsy in whom the risk is very low. The precise manner in which SUDEP is discussed needs to be tailored to the individual patient/family as readiness to learn, ability to learn, psychological, and cultural factors vary widely.

Regrettably, relatively little is known about the best means of patient/family and care provider communications regarding this difficult discussion. One survey of neurologists in the UK indicated that only 26% of physicians routinely discussed SUDEP. In contrast, almost half of epilepsy nurse specialists did so as part of physician directed, patient education. Of note, although expected emotional reactions were frequent, the discussion appeared to increase compliance with medication in the majority of individuals. In summary, education regarding the possibility of death related to seizures should be part of every education plan. The timing of the discussion and emphasis that is given to SUDEP is directly related to relative risk of its occurrence based upon published, high risk factors (e.g. frequent, generalized tonic-clonic seizures). Even in those individuals at minimal risk, the topic should be raised at some point, if only to decrease potential anxiety.

Jeffrey Buchhalter
Phoenix Children's Hospital, Phoenix, AZ, USA.

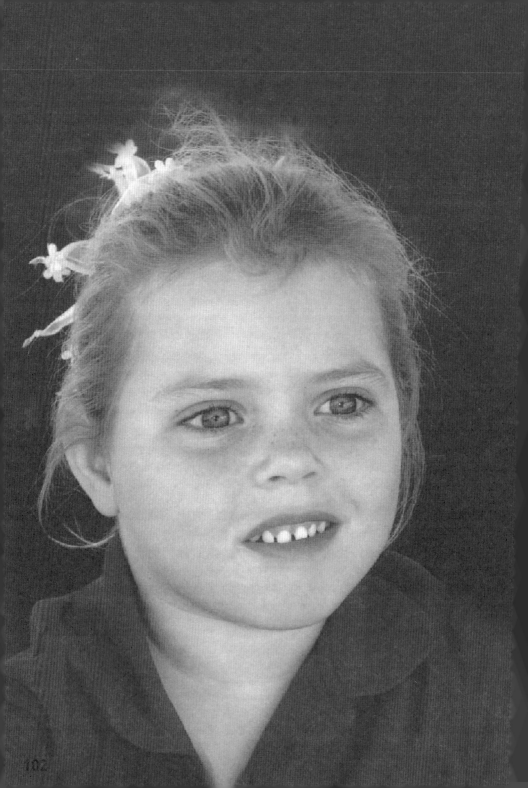

Sophie

Sophie was born a very healthy, happy little girl. She had her first tonic-clonic seizure when she was 6 months old and it lasted 45 minutes. We were discharged from the hospital after a couple of days with a pamphlet about febrile convulsions and told that it was very common for children to have these convulsions up to age 5.

After the next couple of prolonged seizures we had an EEG and were told there was slowing in her brain and what they believed was seizure activity. And then the diagnosis – epilepsy.

The years ahead she battled through seizures, we visited many specialists, had many tests and tried various drugs, and were even involved in a trial of a new drug, but all were of no value and her seizures never slowed down. When Sophie was 3 years old we were told that we may get some seizure control if she had a small piece of her temporal lobe removed. We had no change in Sophie's seizure patterns after surgery. The surgery resulted in us being told she had Dravet's Syndrome, a difficult epilepsy to control.

Sophie plodded along in her life; she was a very happy girl. She went to an early intervention kindergarten and then on to special school. Along our journey we have had mountains of support from family, friends and Sophie's paediatrician. He is a great doctor and all in all a great friend. Nothing was ever sugar-coated, we always knew things were going to be hard for Sophie. I remember being in the hospital and my mum turned to him and said this is a big one John, I'm worried. He turned to us and said it won't be the biggest one I'm afraid!

On our next visit we talked about SUDEP. I always knew that it could happen but the thought of my little girl dying from epilepsy was something I couldn't imagine.

On Monday the 1st of June 2002, I put Sophie to bed as usual, she had her medication, we looked at a book and she listened to her favourite Wiggles song, *Murray Had A Turtle*! She stirred at 1.30am which was nothing unusual and I went to her and put her back to bed. She never woke up. Autopsy results say SUDEP.

Every night when I close my eyes all I see is my beautiful baby . . . gone. She was 7 years old. It's so important to get the SUDEP message out to everyone who has epilepsy in their life. It's heartbreaking to think about but it's necessary to talk about.

Rachel Goss

SUDEP: legal issues

SUDEP is a dreaded and final phenomena which is not infrequent in persons with epilepsy, is poorly understood, sometimes difficult to conclusively confirm, and only questionably preventable. All of these circumstances create a perfect climate for litigious activity.

Litigation involving SUDEP has been initiated in the US over the last 15 years. The primary focus of litigation has employed SUDEP in very different ways. Details of some legal cases are presented in recent chapters by Leestma (2011) and by Wannamaker (2011). Illustrative cases include issues of failure to inform, poor documentation, injury causing epilepsy then SUDEP, and protection of the innocent by sound professional education about epilepsy including SUDEP.

Case 1. A patient discontinued her medication without advice because of side effects. SUDEP occurred. Her long-time physician was sued by her husband who alleged that the physician had failed to advise his wife of the possibility of SUDEP if off medication. At mediation the physician remained steadfast in his position of verbal communication and was dismissed without trial. Careful documentation by the physician may have averted this allegation.

Case 2. A 34 year old woman wanted to become pregnant and was 9 years seizure-free. With counsel of her neurologist a plan of medication withdrawal was nearly complete when SUDEP occurred. Risk of SUDEP was not mentioned in the medical chart. The defense attorney established that the victim had died of SUDEP and also that the cause of SUDEP was unknown. The attorney then argued legally that if the cause of a medical condition is unknown, then the physician cannot be held responsible. The jury verdict was in favor of the physician. Parenthetically, this case would not meet the bar for heightened SUDEP risk (high seizure frequency).

Case 3. A burglar assaulted a woman who resided on a US military reservation. She survived brain injury yet was left with posttraumatic epilepsy. Several years later she died of SUDEP. The assailant had been incarcerated for another crime. He confessed to the burglary in order to obtain sanctuary in another and safer prison. He was unaware of her death. US federal authorities charged the man with murder based on the fact that he induced injury which caused epilepsy and which eventually led to her death. Although convicted of murder, a technicality on appeal reversed the court's conviction. This case brings up extended possibilities when someone is injured and the victim develops epilepsy.

Case 4. A 48 year old woman was found dead in bed at home. Her husband of 30 years was charged with murder by suffocation. She had refractory epilepsy from early childhood. There was no motivation for the husband to murder his wife. The expert for the defense educated the jury that her death could readily be explained by SUDEP. The jury found the husband not guilty.

The future holds widespread recognition of SUDEP amongst patients, families and physicians. In essence, we are already there. Multiple media are replete with references and resources about SUDEP. It is anticipated that the education of patients, families, physicians, and the public may attenuate a rising tide of litigation.

All patients with epilepsy should be provided information about SUDEP and other injurious risks. A physician may reasonably recognize reasons that SUDEP information should not be provided to a specific patient. In either case, the physician is wise to document the action in the records.

A Task Force of the American Epilepsy Society and the Epilepsy Foundation (So et al. 2009) will develop guidelines about how, when and what to say to patients and families about SUDEP. Those guidelines will likely be similar to those of the National Institute for Health and Clinical Excellence (Stokes et al. 2004). Positive and helpful guidelines should facilitate advances in understanding of SUDEP.

The most advantageous patient position is to have an informed and communicative healthcare provider. The safest position for our patients includes both of us being well informed about SUDEP. Hopefully, this guidance will limit future grief and litigation by prevention.

Braxton B. Wannamaker
Clinical Professor
Medical University of South Carolina, Charleston, SA, USA.

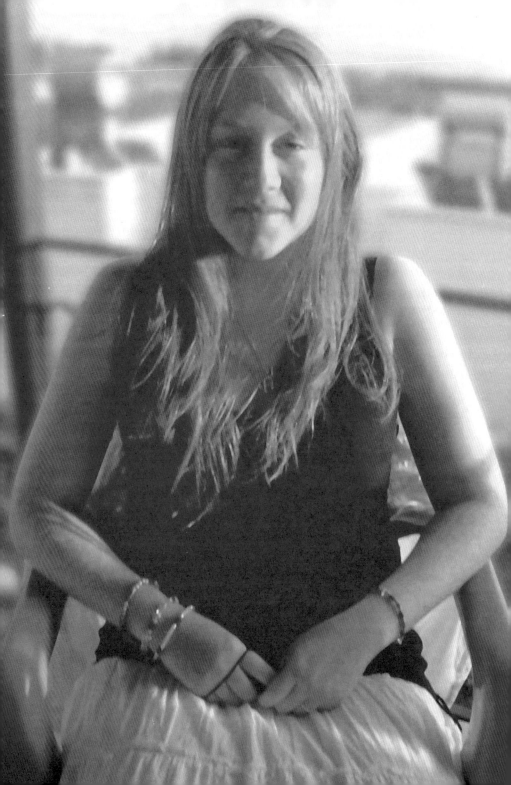

Erin

I could talk all day about Erin, telling you how beautiful, clever, kind, caring, popular, fun loving, annoying, and special she was. Due to leave home for university, she was diagnosed with tonic-clonic seizures and put on antiepileptic medication following a nocturnal seizure. I remember the neurologist saying 'this will just be a minor nuisance in Erin's life'. Five months later she had a second review when her medication was reduced because Erin was worried about putting on weight and tiredness.

Erin was 19 when she died in her sleep some six weeks after starting university. She was getting used to university life. She was not taking her medication as she should have been; she was missing doses.

I first heard of SUDEP when it appeared on Erin's death certificate. The hospital had not contacted us and we had to search the internet for death in epilepsy and discover what SUDEP was. We rang the neurologist and told him we were coming to see him. When asked, he explained that his practice was not to routinely inform about SUDEP because he did not want to cause distress and there was nothing Erin could have done.

We believed that Erin would have taken her condition more seriously, taken her medication properly and we could have supported her. At least she would have had the chance to. The risk might have been remote but it was the most serious risk she faced. Scottish National guidelines recommend SUDEP as essential information for people with epilepsy and in 2002 a judge determined in the Findlay Fatal Accident Inquiry that people with epilepsy should be told, unless there was a good reason not to.

Driven by the attitude of the neurologist, I decided to challenge. A complaint to the hospital was dismissed. I contacted the Scottish Public Services Ombudsman. Two years later the Ombudsman's final report concluded that as there was no record of the decision not to tell Erin, and because no written information was provided, the hospital had failed to provide patient-centred care. She wrote to the government urgently recommending research into communication about SUDEP – this is now being funded.

Independently, the Scottish Government ordered a Fatal Accident Inquiry (FAI) into Erin's death and into the death of another young woman, Christina, who also died from SUDEP. The two Inquiries which have been joined together have involved evidence taking over many months and will report during 2011.

I feel we have achieved what we set out to do; the hospital has recruited a specialist nurse and is providing written information. Regardless of the outcome of the FAI, we have been listened to and the arguments have been carefully considered by independent professionals. This has taken years now and at great personal cost to our family. It was not a matter of courage or bravery, it was about the need to make sense of what happened. As time passed I also came to appreciate that in her name, changes could come about that would mean that Erin did not die for nothing.

Janet Casey

107

SUDEP: the needs of the bereaved

Bereavement affects people uniquely, but there is evidence that while sudden bereavement can complicate grieving, early intervention can reduce associated morbidity (Yates, Ellison & McGuiness 1990).

People who have experienced a sudden traumatic loss such as SUDEP acknowledge that on occasions, the pain can overwhelm. This pain coupled with lack of SUDEP awareness in the community leaves people feeling uncared-for and isolated. Systems are often not in place to prevent painful situations such as patient appointment letters being sent to the bereaved or a home being treated as a crime scene investigation.

During the early stages of bereavement, counsellors may feel that it is too soon for bereavement counselling. However, people who feel the need for help may be assisted through bereavement support. *I just can't talk to anybody about this because they say it is too soon. But it's eating me away – not knowing what to do next* (bereaved parent).

Although in the UK Epilepsy Bereaved is listed by the Government as the specialist organization to support people affected by SUDEP, 80% of contacts result from web searches by the bereaved.

Data from the UK supports the demand for, and value of, a specialist service. During the 12 months ending March 2011 Epilepsy Bereaved responded to 79 newly bereaved people and 1382 calls from a total of 1116 bereaved families. The confidential, caller-led service is run by two bereavement counsellors who are trained to understand the specific needs of those bereaved by an epilepsy related death and the post death procedures and institutions that they encounter. A particular feature of sudden death is the overwhelming need to understand. Typical questions are: Could I have done anything? Did they suffer? Would they have been calling for me? Why didn't they tell me this could happen? Did they suffocate? Would an alarm have helped? The service is supported by a panel of SUDEP experts and offers information resources on epilepsy mortality.

Twenty percent of calls are more complex and in these situations SUDEP experts may be asked to review questions from families regarding the post-mortem or events leading up to the death, although to maintain confidentiality all clinical notes are anonymized. As part of the grieving process there is often anger. Epilepsy Bereaved staff are trained not to give any view but to listen. Very few go on to seek further inquiry. This is most likely when solicitors are instructed before contact is made with the charity.

For the newly bereaved there often appears to be no respite, no way out of the dark place that they find themselves in – until they find someone who has been there too. There is frequently a bond to be found existing between those who have lost someone of a similar age or in similar circumstances.

Epilepsy Bereaved holds meetings throughout the UK for those affected by an epilepsy-related death to come together for mutual support in a safe environment. It provides opportunities for those who wish to channel their grief in a positive way to explore ways in which they can engage with the work of the charity. During the year ended March 2011, 15% of our families chose to be active in our work, by raising awareness and using their story to influence change, with 80 families participating in research interviews. A national SUDEP memorial service is held every three years.

Led by the changing needs of our members, during 2011 Epilepsy Bereaved will train and support 10 active supporters to become regional ambassadors. The charity is also piloting a telephone counselling service for people unable to access a local service who would benefit from a confidential space where people can explore their feelings and learn coping strategies to help them in their day-to-day lives.

Karen Osland
Support and Liaison Manager
Epilepsy Bereaved, UK.

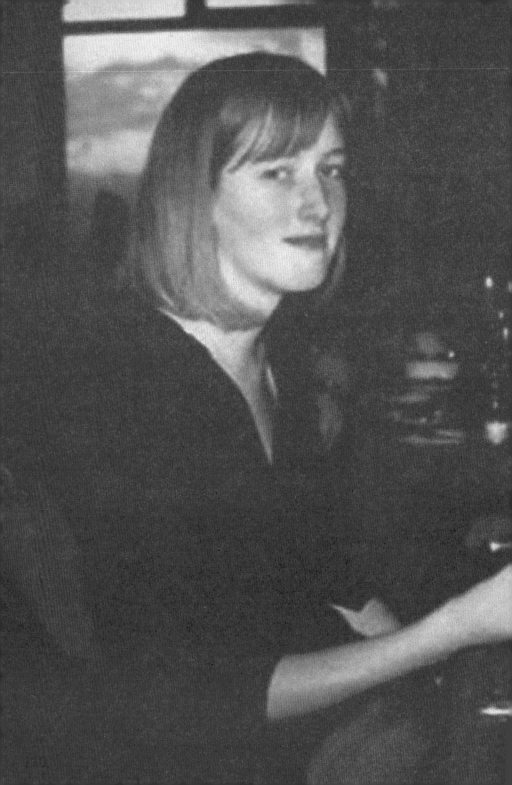

Eve

Eve, the youngest of our two daughters, died aged 21 in 2005 whilst studying Radio & TV Production at Staffordshire University. We thought she had her whole life ahead of her. She had been diagnosed when she was 13 years old; we knew nothing of SUDEP.

Eve was quiet and quite reserved, very much a listener, which made her very easy going. Never any bother, liking nothing better than any excuse to get her duvet down and watch TV, she was very much a home-bird. Eve was obsessed with the Brownies, she always took it very seriously, working hard and determinedly to earn her badges. She loved helping the younger Brownies, mothering them on Brownie camp holidays.

As a young adult she found a new found interest in film. We always said films were entertainment, but to Eve they were so much more. Explaining to 'the parentals' (as she called us) how important they were.

Her friendship base was the same until university where she met an extended family; we are still friends with them. Eve had many friends and was enjoying the independence that came with university life. Her best friend Steph loves keeping in contact with us. She once said; "we are the closest thing to Eve that she has".

Eve was the type of girl who touched many people's lives.

On the 15th October – Eve's birthday, we attended an Epilepsy Bereaved meeting in Liverpool. It was as if fate guided us there, we could be nowhere else. We met others who knew a little of how we felt and who understood the depth of our loss – let's face it loosing a child doesn't get much worse

Afterwards we felt a new sense of purpose; we had decided to campaign to try and secure an epilepsy specialist nurse in our area. We needed to feel that Eve didn't die in vain and felt this would give us a focus and help us in our most difficult journey. It was an uphill struggle, but in 2006 our efforts paid off and the nurse was appointed. The campaign brought with it lots of emotions, but we realize that every single set back, disappointment, heartache and frustration was worth it.

I am 6 years down the line now, and feel that I am ready to pass on my experience and insight to others. I am currently looking to becoming an ambassador for EB and I see raising awareness of the risks of epilepsy as a lifelong commitment.

Eve didn't survive to "make a difference" in her adult life, but I can do it for her.

Denise Brown

SUDEP: clinical practice

There are no studies assessing the effectiveness of any particular measure to prevent SUDEP, and such studies of course would be difficult to carry out. However, a number of clinical features have been identified which increase the risk of SUDEP, and any measures which can minimise the risk of these features in clinical practice are very likely to reduce the incidence of SUDEP. As SUDEP in most cases occurs in the aftermath of a generalized convulsive seizure and as a high frequency of convulsive seizures is the most important risk factor, measures aimed at lowering the frequency of convulsive seizures are the most important. Other factors include poor compliance, potential risks of certain drugs, switching drugs, seizures at night, apnea or cardiac rhythm changes during seizures (Shorvon & Tomson, 2011).

Antiepileptic and other drugs: The association between antiepileptic drug therapy and SUDEP is complicated. It is likely that any drug therapy which reduces the frequency of convulsive seizures will reduce the incidence of SUDEP, and indeed, one published case control study showed that the absence of treatment increased the risk of SUDEP 21.7 fold when compared to therapy with one or two antiepileptic drugs (Langan, Nashef & Sander 2005). However, other studies have not shown a statistically significant effect. Periods of non-adherence with therapy have also been associated with an increased risk of SUDEP (Cramer, Glassman & Rienzi 2002, Téllez-Zenteno, Ronquillo & Wiebe 2005, Williams et al. 2006, Monté et al. 2007, Faught et al. 2008). Similarly, frequent changes in therapy have been shown to be associated with an increased risk of SUDEP (Nilsson et al. 1999).

It has also been suggested that antiepileptic drug therapy could increase the risk of SUDEP, through effects on cardiac conduction. Most studies have focused on the sodium-channel drugs carbamazepine and lamotrigine, and there is some evidence that both are rarely a cause of fatal cardiac arrhythmias. However, large studies have generally not shown any association with any particular therapy and there is currently no definitive evidence to suggest that any particular antiepileptic drug should be avoided. Some antipsychotics and other drugs can prolong the QT-interval and have caused sudden cardiac death (Hancox & Witchel 2000) but whether this is a mechanism of SUDEP is not known.

Epilepsy surgery: If epilepsy surgery successfully reduces the frequency of generalized tonic-clonic seizures, it would be expected to lower the risk of SUDEP. Some studies have demonstrated this (Annegers et al. 2000, Nilsson et al. 2003, Salanova, Markand & Worth 2005, Sperling et al. 2005, Jehi 2010).

Vagal nerve stimulation: There has been concern about the risk that vagal nerve stimulation might induce bradycardia or cardiac arrest, and in occasional patients, a bradycardia or asystole is induced. However, a review of a cohort of 1,819 individuals partially funded by the manufacturers of the device (3,176, person-years from implantation) revealed only 25 deaths and the authors considered that this was no higher than rates previously reported in other chronic epilepsy populations (Annegers et al. 2000).

Cardiac pacing as a preventative measure: Ictal bradycardia is common (Rugg-Gunn et al. 2004) and might increase the risk of SUDEP (So & Sperling 2007; Schuele et al. 2008). In patients with a demonstrated marked ictal cardiac arrhythmia cardiac pacing is commonly recommended as a preventative measure against SUDEP (Lim, Lim & Wilder-Smith 2000, Rossetti et al. 2005, Schuele, Bermeo et al. 2007). It has been also suggested that in complex partial seizures in which there is sudden loss of tone (causing a 'drop attack'), this symptom might indicate ictal asystole, and that these patients are at particular risk of SUDEP. Cardiac monitoring, with a view to pacing should be considered in patients with this ictal feature (Rossetti et al. 2005, Schuele, Bermeo et al. 2007).

General advice to minimise the risk of SUDEP:

■ **Reduction of tonic-clonic seizures**: Tonic-clonic seizures should be viewed as potentially lethal events and their occurrence taken very seriously. Any measures which reduce these are likely to reduce the risk of seizures. Thus, advice should be given to patients about lifestyle issues, avoiding precipitants (alcohol, sleep deprivation etc) and also about compliance with medication.

■ **Drug changes**: These should be made cautiously. If switching medication, it is usually best to introduce the new drug before withdrawing the old drug. The changes should staged in a gradual fashion. The patients should have access to immediate advice in the event of worsening seizures during the switch over period - this is a particularly hazardous period from the point of view of SUDEP.

- **Supervision at night**: Supervision at night should be considered when there is a risk of uncontrolled tonic-clonic seizures. This of course needs to be balanced against the penalties of intrusive monitoring.

- **Choice of drugs**: Caution should be applied to the use of drugs which have potential cardio-respiratory adverse effects.

- **Cardio-respiratory warning signs**: Special attention should be paid to prolonged tonic-clonic seizures, seizures with marked cyanosis, seizures with periods of severe bradycardia or apnea, seizures with marked atonia (drop attackes) in the presence of pre-existing cardiac or respiratory impairment. In these patients, cardiac pacing considered if there is a risk of severe arrhythmia.

- **Supervision of a seizure**: It is important to attend a patient after a generalized convulsive seizure until full consciousness is restored. This is especially important if emergency drug therapy has been given which can depress respiration. The attendant should be aware of the risk of cardiac or respiratory arrest and be ready, wherever possible, to institute emergency measures. The emergency services should be called in any seizure occurring in the community in which there is considered to be a high risk of cardio-respiratory depression. Proper supervision will also help avoid non-SUDEP deaths caused by accidental injury or aspiration of vomit for instance.

- **Counselling on the risks**: Decisions about lifestyle and therapy are the perogative of the patient. The physician's role is to provide a risk .v. benefit analysis. The risks of SUDEP should be considered in formulating such advice.

Simon Shorvon
Professor of Clinical Neurology
UCL Institute of Neurology, London, UK.

Part 4.

facing the challenges

Standing up for epilepsy

Epilepsy is not a benign disease, epilepsy kills! Each year, in Europe, a so-called developed part of the world, there are 13,000 deaths, 40% of which could be prevented with proper access to correct diagnosis and treatment.

Through the centuries, there were many misconceptions about the condition, based on the culture of a particular era or place in the world. As Rajendra Kale said: 'The history of epilepsy can be summarized as 4,000 years of ignorance, superstition and stigma, followed by 100 years of knowledge, superstition and stigma' (Kale 1997).

Dr. Gro Harlem Brundtland (2002), (Director General WHO 1998-2003) said at the 2nd launch of the Global Campaign in 2001: 'Around fifty million people suffer from epilepsy. Many of them suffer silently. Many of them suffer alone. Beyond the suffering and beyond the absence of care lie the frontiers of stigma, shame, exclusion and, more often than we care to know, death.'

Despite these obvious burdens, however, in recent decades, epilepsy has been painted as a disorder that can be treated and, if that treatment is available, people with epilepsy can live happily ever after…but do they?

Which raises the question: What is epilepsy? Epilepsy is the world's most common brain disorder, affecting 50 million people worldwide, 85% of whom live in developing countries. Epilepsy is a global problem affecting all ages, races, and social classes. It imposes enormous physical, psychological, social and economic burdens on individuals, families and countries, due to misunderstanding, fear and stigma. Globally: 250,000,000 people have one seizure in a life time; 2,500,000 new cases of epilepsy occur each year; 70% of people with epilepsy could be seizure-free with (cheap) treatment; and 80% of people with epilepsy do not receive a proper diagnosis and are not properly treated.

The solutions to these problems are too complex to be solved by individual organizations. Therefore, the three leading international organizations – the International League Against Epilepsy (ILAE), the International Bureau for Epilepsy (IBE), and the World Health Organization (WHO) – have joined forces in the Global Campaign Against Epilepsy (GCAE) to bring epilepsy 'out of the shadows'. The Campaign aims to assist governments worldwide to ensure that the diagnosis, treatment, prevention and social acceptability of epilepsy are improved. The strategy has two parallel tracks: raising awareness and understanding of epilepsy; and supporting governments to identify the needs and to promote education, research, training, prevention, treatment and care services. The Campaign's objective is to ensure that epilepsy is on the health and development agenda and implement cost-effective care.

Over 100 countries have developed Campaign activities. IBE, ILAE and WHO collaboration has built a framework for global, regional and national action to raise awareness and diminish the treatment gap. However, epilepsy continues to take its toll; people with epilepsy are often stigmatized, which discourages them from seeking the diagnosis and care they require.

Mortality rates among people with epilepsy are two to three times higher than in the general population. An estimated 40% of all epilepsy-related deaths are SUDEPs. The cause of SUDEP remains unknown and awareness of risk factors is very low. WHO is aware of this high mortality and one of its Collaborating Centres, Stichting Epilepsie Instellinjgen Nederland (SEIN) is conducting a systematic review on the mortality of epilepsy and its temporal trends. Mortality studies are taking place in Georgia, China and the UK ('Epilepsy must become a higher priority in Europe' 2010).

However, research badly needs more funding. Research into the mortality of epilepsy and other aspects of epilepsy is vital in order to improve our understanding and ultimately improve patient care. Cure and prevention of epilepsy are still distant goals, but in the meantime many people with epilepsy are needlessly struggling with poor health, prejudice and death.

Epilepsy must be given a higher priority by governments, policymakers, healthcare professionals, and communities, within all countries. Epilepsy Advocacy Europe (EAE) is a joint taskforce set up by the ILAE and IBE with its mission to enhance public awareness and to support research in epilepsy in Europe. EAE seeks to make epilepsy a priority in political and research establishments across Europe. Its motto is: 'Stand up for Epilepsy'

The potential for seizure control in many patients should not be taken as a sign that epilepsy is not important. Thus, using the EAE's motto: 'let's stand up for epilepsy,' the 50 million people with epilepsy deserve better.

Hanneke M. de Boer
Senior Officer International Contacts//Research Departmental Co-ordinator
SEIN – Epilepsy Institute in the Netherlands.

Australia

When *Sudden Unexpected Death in Epilepsy: a global conversation* was published in 2005 we reflected on advancements in SUDEP awareness and action in the previous decade, whilst acknowledging that many challenges remained. Good things have happened in Australia since 2005 but change is slow. Despite our best efforts, six years on, families are still discovering SUDEP through the death of a loved one. In 2010 one bereaved family felt so frustrated by what they perceived as a lack of community awareness that they created their own support organisation. This suggests that while celebrating improvements in epilepsy care, we need to continually reflect on what we can improve.

Memorial services continue to be held every second year, as they have for ten years, with the encouragement of bereaved families. The families are generous in their support of any publicity initiatives and are willing to speak with the media. This has resulted in articles in major newspapers, TV news and current affairs reports, and participation in a TV documentary examining the work of the Victorian Institute of Forensic Medicine.

In 2008, we launched the Parliamentary Friends of Epilepsy group at Parliament House Canberra. The topic of the meeting was SUDEP and several bereaved parents were invited to speak. The formation of this link to national government is a wonderful opportunity to highlight the needs of people with epilepsy, including the risks of epilepsy-related death. In 2009 the Parliamentary Friends of Epilepsy held an informal inquiry into the impact of epilepsy in Australia and a submission, including SUDEP data, was put forward by the Joint Epilepsy Council of Australia (JECA).

We continue to nurture international links. An Epilepsy Bereaved (UK) representative participated with us in SUDEP sessions at the 8th Asian and Oceanian Epilepsy Congress in Melbourne in 2010. We have developed links with organizations in North America, and were invited to attend the SUDEP meeting at the National Institute of Health in Washington in 2008.

Looking to the future, Epilepsy Australia has created the *Reducing Epilepsy Deaths (RED)* project. The aim is to clarify current understanding of epilepsy-related death in Australia (and the world), and to map the direction of our future work. Bereaved families have always been the backbone of our activites and consideration is being given to how best to support their ongoing participation. To date, SUDEP projects have struggled for funding, and the current work is being funded by a small SUDEP education and research fund established by Epilepsy Australia. However, the vision of this project is that by taking time to gather data to make a strong, clear case for the necessary strategies, our work will become more effective and also more attractive to funding bodies.

Epilepsy deaths are strongly associated with seizures and discussions of reducing epilepsy deaths always lead back to the need for quality care. In the UK, it is the conversation regarding epilepsy-related deaths that has done more than anything else to bring about changes in health care policies affecting epilepsy. In Australia the RED project has identified GPs as a key link in the epilepsy care chain and an online GP survey is underway to guide resource development. The RED project is strengthened by the fact that this survey is being carried out in collaboration with our colleagues at Epilepsy New Zealand.

One fundamental problem in attracting resources and support for SUDEP is the lack of reliable data. Therefore as part of the RED project a successful application was made to the National Coronial Information Service (NCIS) to instigate an examination of all epilepsy-related deaths recorded in the system for the past 10 years. This is a unique project with the potential to reveal informative data regarding the circumstances of epilepsy-related deaths. The knowledge gained will be of value in Australia, and also internationally.

The ultimate aim of all our work is a reduction of epilepsy-related deaths and enhanced quality of life for people with epilepsy

Rosemary Panelli & Denise Chapman

South East Asia

There is very limited data on SUDEP in South East Asia. In rural Laos, high mortality rates were reported during a community-based phenobarbital program. Six of the 53 patients (11%) died during the 2-year study (drowning 2, burns 1, fall 1, sudden unspecified cause 2)(Tran et al. 2006, Tran et al. 2008). For Asia generally, there are reports of high mortality among epilepsy patients (Tan 2007) with injury as the major cause of death reported in rural areas. Ding et al. (2006) noted 35 deaths among 2,455 people with epilepsy in rural China, but only one case (2.9%) was attributed to SUDEP. The main cause of death was accidental or other causes of injury (including self-inflicted injury) in 13 people (37%), (drowning 6, suicide 4, poisoning 2, road traffic accidents 1). The mortality in epilepsy was reported as 7.63 per 100,000 population per year in Kolkata, India (Banerjee et al. 2010) and 0.5 per 100,000 in Singapore (Puvanendran 1993), but the cause of death was not specified in these reports. In contrast to the rural regions, Taiwan reported 18.8% of the epilepsy mortality as due to SUDEP, with a standard mortality ratio (SMR) of 3.47 (Chen et al. 2005)

Novel findings in relation to SUDEP have been identified by researchers in Asia, although they were working with a limited number of patients and few resources. Teh et al. (2007), from Malaysia reported a significant shorter mean QT interval corrected for heart rate (QTc) in epilepsy patients as compared to controls (0.401 +/- 0.027s vs. 0.420 +/- 0.027s, p<0.0005). Shortening of QT indicates pathological cardiac repolarization, which is a known risk of sudden cardiac death. (Surges et al. 2010) In Taiwan, Harnod et al. (2009) reported a lower mean heart rate interval and a lower high frequency power in patients with frontal lobe epilepsy using frequency-domain analysis of heart rate variability. The author concluded that faster heart rates, attributed to lower parasympathetic drive, might contribute to the higher incidence of sudden death that is seen in this group of patients.

With regard to medical statements and practice, as far as we are aware, there is no regional initiative to promote research and awareness of SUDEP in South East Asia, or Asia generally. As for the effort by the individual countries, in Malaysia the local consensus guideline has included a section on SUDEP to raise the awareness of general practitioners. There is also inclusion of SUDEP in the patient drug information leaflets. It can be concluded that there should be more attention to SUDEP in neurology practice throughout the region.

In conclusion there is very limited data on mortality generally, and SUDEP in particular, in South East Asia. But taking Asia as a whole there are indications that mortality in epilepsy is significantly increased as compared to the general population. Accidental injury is the major cause of death, and SUDEP is also a significant cause of mortality. There is a need to have better data collection on epilepsy mortality including SUDEP in South East Asia. There is also a need to promote greater awareness of SUDEP in the medical practice of the region.

Kheng-Seang Lim and Chong-Tin Tan
Division of Neurology
Department of Medicine
University of Malaya, Kuala Lumpur, Malaysia.

Taiwan

In Taiwan, when studying the cause of the death in persons with epilepsy, it is convenient to use the death certificate system from the Department of Health. A death certificate is a document issued by a government official and requires a doctor to record the etiology for the death, and to declare the date, location and cause of a person's death.

If the patient is a Taiwanese citizen with an ID card, the death can be identified through the system correctly for the following reasons: it is mandatory for local household registration offices to submit standardized certificates of each death to the Department of Health; residents are required to register all birth, death, marriage, divorce, and migration events with the household registration offices; registered household information is checked annually through a home-visit interview by the registration office; and the record linkage is straightforward because the Death Certification System uses the national ID number, which is unique for each resident of Taiwan.

The major problem for this system is how the doctors code the etiology for the death. In most circumstances, the decision will be clear. For example, if the person had an episode of status epilepticus with mortality, the etiology of the death could be respiratory failure and the leading cause would be status epilepticus. If the person died from a traffic accident, the etiology for the death could be tricky. Our law bans the driving privilege for people with epilepsy. If a person with epilepsy has a fatal traffic accident, the family will probably hide the history of epilepsy to avoid the penalty. It will be hard to know the true reason for the death unless the person was seen to have a seizure during the traffic accident.

It's not easy to get an autopsy to study the possible cause of death. Unless an autopsy is required by court order when the death is the result of a criminal act or there is uncertainty as to the cause of death, the request for an autopsy is usually rejected by the family. To have a whole, intact, and undamaged body is our culture's chief concern for the bereaved family. Even though the name 'epilepsy' still horrifies many in our culture, when a person with epilepsy dies the family will admit to the police officer that the person had epilepsy and that the cause of the unexpected death was probably a seizure, so that he will be inclined to classify the case as a natural death or death from the disease.

In the past few years our fellow researchers have used this national death certificate system to study the cause of epilepsy-related death in Taiwan. The major etiologies recorded for the deaths were status epilepticus and traffic accidents. Suicide and SUDEP were also recorded. Weaknesses in the death certificate reporting were noted and researchers concluded that a long-term cohort study is needed to understand the true incidence of SUDEP.

Around 300 persons with epilepsy are regularly followed up in my clinic and I have encountered two true SUDEP cases. Both of them were male; one was 35 years old and the other was 27 years old. Both were found dead in the morning by their family. The causes of the death were unknown. The 35 year old man had a history of partial seizures with secondary generalization. He took medication regularly, but at the time of his death he had stopped his medication because he was going to have surgery. An autopsy was not done. The 27 year old man had a generalized epilepsy syndrome. He had ceased his medication for six months due to a remission of seizures for more than 2 years. He was found dead in the morning by his sister. An autopsy was also not done. A 30 year old woman who came to the clinic with a syncopal episode reported that her sister had died suddenly because of seizures. However, investigation of the syncope revealed that the family of the women had long QT syndrome. The patient was transferred to a cardiologist and the follow up was fine. Her sister's death may have been miscoded.

The true incidence and etiology for SUDEP needs to be established through a long-term cohort study. However, the death certificate is still a useful guide for the mortality rate for the persons with epilepsy in our society.

Shung-Lon Lai
Department of Neurology
Kaohsiung Chang-Gung Memorial Hospital
Chang-Gung University, College of Medicine, Kaohsiung, Taiwan.

Malta

Malta is a small island state and a member of the European Union, centrally located in Mediterranean sea. The population is just over 400,000 and preliminary studies indicate that the incidence of epilepsy in Malta (4000 persons or just under 1% of the population) is similar to that in Europe. The local IBE association, the Caritas Malta Epilepsy Association, was set up in 1996 and became affiliated to IBE in 1999. The Association is for persons with epilepsy and their families. It aims to promote education and local awareness about epilepsy, especially because of the stigma suffered by people with this condition socially and in the workplace. Our campaign is aimed at the continual improvement of health care services. Our goal is for the management and social acceptance of epilepsy, to reflect the fact that it is a serious, yet treatable, brain disorder.

Raising public and professional awareness and dispelling myths about epilepsy is one of our key objectives since there is still a great deal of stigma and discrimination in Malta. The emphasis over the past few years has been on a promotional and educational campaign of the various aspects of epilepsy in the Maltese language. Caritas Malta Epilepsy Association now lists over 300 members and its conferences regularly attract over 250 participants.

The 9th European Epilepsy & Society Conference, held in Malta 2004, was the first European conference to have SUDEP on its agenda, and included personal experiences of SUDEP across Europe. However, SUDEP is still an unknown entity here in Malta and is rarely addressed either in the Association's meetings or in its biannual conferences. There is also a general lack of awareness of SUDEP among Maltese people with epilepsy, their carers, and their relatives.

Data obtained from the Health Information and Research Department in the Ministry of Health indicates that between 2000-2009 there were a total of 29 deaths in Malta, which were listed in the UCD code as being related to epilepsy. One death was listed as being due to generalized idiopathic epilepsy and epileptic syndromes, 18 deaths were classified as epilepsy (unspecified), while in 9 deaths the cause was listed as being due to status epilepticus. However, no more information is available and so far no research has been undertaken locally in this regard.

The Caritas Malta Epilepsy Association organizes various educational and outreach activities emphasizing examples of good practice which will help to improve seizure control and thus reduce unexpected deaths from epilepsy. One of the recent outreach activities in March 2011 was the organization of an Epilepsy Day on campus at the University of Malta. Participants included Malta Pharmaceutical Student Association, Malta Medical Student Association and Malta Association of Dental Students in conjunction with the Caritas and Department of Clinical Pharmacology and Therapeutics. The students prepared a leaflet which described appropriate first aid in various types of epilepsies, yet SUDEP was not covered in this leaflet.

There is a long way to go until SUDEP is discussed openly among the epilepsy community in Malta. The subject is still taboo in many spheres and some people with epilepsy and their families do not acknowledge it as being a problem. Education and awareness raising on SUDEP is very important and these have a key role to play in reducing the lack of understanding of this important consequence of epilepsy.

Janet Mifsud
Advisor, Caritas Malta Epilepsy Association, Malta.

China

One percent of people in the world have epilepsy, over 80% of whom live in developing countries. It is estimated that 9,000,000 people have epilepsy in China, increasing by 450,000 newly diagnosed patients annually. Up to two thirds of these people live in rural areas and do not receive regular treatment mainly because of difficulties with the treatment infrastructure and the availability of suitable drugs. People with epilepsy have increased risk of premature death compared with the general population. However, the extent and nature of this risk, especially SUDEP, has not been sufficiently examined in China.

In late 1980's, 120 patients with epilepsy were recruited in the 'Community Control of Epilepsy Project' in China. Thirteen patients were found to have died during the 5-year follow-up. Among the 13 deceased, two (15.4%) might be categorized as SUDEP (Wang & Li 1993). Clinical and pathological findings in 7 SUDEP cases were reported by Wang et al. (2004). Besides having edema of brain and lung, some of the deceased patients had a reduction of neurons and an increase of gliocytes. Neoplasms or injuries in the brain were not found. All seven patients died during generalized tonic-clonic seizures; two in sleep. Four of them had agitation or fright before death.

In 1997 the World Health Organization (WHO), in cooperation with the International League against Epilepsy (ILAE) and the International Bureau for Epilepsy (IBE), launched the Global Campaign Against Epilepsy in an attempt to bring epilepsy 'out of the shadows' and to improve the treatment of people with epilepsy in resource-poor countries. One demonstration project, 'Epilepsy Management at Primary Health Level' (EMPHL), under the auspices of the WHO and the Ministry of Health of China, was implemented in rural areas in six non-contiguous provinces of China. The EMPHL protocol used strict follow-up and management procedures to follow and assess mortality in people with epilepsy in rural China. During follow-up local primary-care physicians recorded demographic data and a putative cause of death for any patient who died. Cause of death was attributed on clinical grounds and verbal autopsy. Specialists and the principal investigators in each study area gathered information about cause of death through interviews with relatives or local village physicians. Death certificates were also used for confirmation of the cause of death.

By June 2004, the first follow-up wave (median follow-up time of 25 months) found 35 deaths among 2,455 people with epilepsy. The Standardized Mortality Ratio (SMR) was 3.9 (95% CI: 3.8-3.9). Patients aged 15-29 years had higher mortality ratios than did those in other age-groups, with SMRs exceeding 23. The main cause of death was accidental or as a result of injury. In one third of patients, death was attributed to hemorrhagic or ischemic stroke, and in two people death was attributed to pneumonia. In one patient death was attributed to SUDEP after a negative post mortem examination, while in three patients the cause of death was not attributed because of lack of information (Ding et al. 2006). By December 2008, the second follow-up wave (median follow-up time of 6.5 years) found 203 deaths in the patient cohort. Among these 203 deceased people with epilepsy, 2 died of SUDEP and 10 died of uncertain cause with inadequate information (unpublished data).

Compared to western countries, SUDEP is rarely reported in people with epilepsy in China. The main reasons might be the lack of knowledge of SUDEP in Chinese physicians and the lack of post mortem examinations to determine SUDEP. Another reason could be that most Chinese patients usually sleep with their carers and this may be good for detecting and taking care of seizures during sleep. If this is the case there will be a glimmer of hope to prevent SUDEP. Further scientific research and education programs are urgently needed in China to face the challenge of SUDEP.

Ding Ding
Institute of Neurology, Fu Dan University, China
WHO Collaborating Center for Research and Training in Neurosciences
China Association Against Epilepsy.

Scotland

Epilepsy Scotland's commitment to raising awareness of SUDEP is as strong as ever. There is no doubt it is an extremely emotive subject with a great disparity of opinion as to how accessible the information about SUDEP should be and when it should be given. As the lead non-government organization in Scotland with an increasingly high profile, we continue an open dialogue with the politicians, policy makers and the media with regards to SUDEP. In addition we feel our work with the Scottish Parliament's Cross Party Group and the Managed Clinical Networks for epilepsy will ensure consistently high quality information on SUDEP is available to all.

In Scotland there is a lack of post mortem evidence to accurately show how many deaths are attributable to SUDEP. Deaths in Scotland are coded using the International Statistical Classification of Diseases and Related Health Problems (ICD-10). SUDEP is coded as 'epilepsy, unspecified' which may be SUDEP – or could be one of many other epilepsy-related causes that have not been specified. However, research shows that the overall incidence of SUDEP is 1:1000 people with epilepsy. In Scotland this would translate as 40 deaths a year.

The risk of SUDEP is often not disclosed to people with epilepsy and the reasons given for that are that the risk of death is small and the possible distress such disclosure may cause. Research conducted by Morton, Richardson and Duncan (2006); showed that of 387 UK neurologists – 5% discussed SUDEP with all patients and 26% discussed SUDEP with the majority. Information was more likely to be given if a patient asked for it, or they had known risk factors.

Although the risk is small and the information may cause some distress to individuals, Epilepsy Scotland believes that people with epilepsy should be informed of all aspects of their condition. Studies have identified some possible risk factors associated with SUDEP. Knowledge of these risks may determine behaviour with regard to treatment concordance, general self-management of their condition and the use of additional safety measures; for example, the use of seizure alarms, which may reduce risk for those experiencing nocturnal seizures. In addition, thought and consideration must be given to those who are left with the loss of someone as a result of SUDEP. The natural distress caused by the loss of a loved one may be exacerbated by feelings of guilt (possibly thought to be misplaced by some) for not taking adequate precautions in order to avoid SUDEP.

The Scottish Government has commissioned Epilepsy Scotland to research the information needs of people with epilepsy regarding SUDEP. Epilepsy Scotland has started the process of planning the research and designing the study with potential partners. The research aims to identify at what point post diagnosis, individuals would prefer to receive information on SUDEP and in what form (printed information, one to one counselling or a combination). Equally important is to identify from whom they would prefer to receive that information – their consultant or an epilepsy specialist nurse.

Epilepsy Scotland is hopeful the results of this research will help to support healthcare professionals in the vital process of information sharing with their patients regarding SUDEP. We aim to produce a best practice guide using input from those who understand their information needs better than anyone else – people living with epilepsy.

Lesslie Young
Executive Officer, Epilepsy Scotland.

Africa

In Africa, epidemiological research has demonstrated a wide range of epilepsy prevalence rates from 0.9 to 43 ‰ (Jallon 1997). However studies about death among people with epilepsy are very rare and no specific report on sudden death has been published in Africa.

In Kenya, a two-year community-based investigation revealed that 3.5 % of the deaths of individuals over the age of 5 occurred to people with epilepsy. Of these deaths 77 % were thought to have occurred whilst the patient was in status epilepticus (Snow et al. 1994).

In Africa, the reported causes of epilepsy-related deaths are usually: status epilepticus; drowning; burns; and non-assistance because of a belief that seizures are a "contagious disease". More than 50% patients die during or after a seizure (Diop et al. 2003, Diop et al. 2005).

Epilepsy-related deaths are also associated with a lack of drug supply due to economic reasons or non-availability. It is easy to guess that hundreds of people with epilepsy are silently dying from SUDEP in Africa, far from the cities and university hospitals statistics.

In rural Tanzania, patients with epilepsy showed an increased mortality rate, which was twice that of the general population of similar age (Jilek-Aall & Rwiza 1992). In Ethiopia, during a period of 2 years, eight persons died of status epilepticus and one from severe burns as a result of falling into a domestic fire during a seizure (Tekle-Haimanot, Forsgren & Ekstedt 1997).

It is estimated that 80-90% of patients with epilepsy in Africa do not receive adequate medical treatment (Diop et al. 2004, Meinardi et al. 2001).

Many factors cause the high rate of epilepsy in the country: the high incidence of infectious diseases; the poor quality of maternal infant care in this low socio-economic country; consanguineous marriages; and delayed diagnosis and management of tumors and traumatic causes (Diop et al. 2004). Poor infrastructure, insufficient availability of drugs, and scarcity of trained medical personnel are relevant factors for this situation (Ndiaye et al. 2000). The majority of people suffering from seizures do not primarily consult a physician. In Sub-Saharan Africa, the ratio is 1 neurologist for 600,000 to 10 million population; the exceptions are North Africa and South Africa with a ratio of 1 neurologist for 250,000 to 400,000 people. In this central part of Africa, there are about 100 EEG machines, 120 CT and 30 MRI scanners available for neurological assessment (Diop et al. 2004).

The main antiepileptic drugs available in the Africa continent are: phenobarbital (prescribed in 65 to 90 %); carbamazepine (5 to 25 %); phenytoin (2 to 25 %); valproate (2 to 8 %) and diazepam for emergency. Very few countries have some of the brand new drugs. The annual prices of drugs range from $25 (for phenobarbital) to $300-500 (for carbamazepine and valproate) (Diop et al. 2004).

Some increased epilepsy awareness and advancement in epilepsy management is beginning to occur. This is a result of improved and decentralized epilepsy health care, communication with the community, and education and intensive training of physicians and paramedical staff coordinated by a League against epilepsy. The Leagues also bring together patients, families, health, workers, social workers and volunteers. In some countries videos, leaflets, seizure diaries, training and guidelines books for health personnel, posters and T-shirts for public advertising have been the tools to improve epilepsy awareness and care. In Senegal a weekly epilepsy clinic has been set up in the capital city Dakar. Based on the concept of a 'Caravan for Epilepsy' it consists of a 3-day intervention. There are: meetings with province administrative and health authorities, and local media; a training course with physicians and paramedical staff; meetings with schools, women's associations and social workers; and finally a day for consultations with patients coming from the villages and small cities. A portable EEG machine is available. Information and education programs are also conducted via TV, radio, newspapers, and public conferences. Session are organized with traditional healers to improve collaboration between modern and traditional medical practice, because it has been found that 88% of patients with epilepsy combine traditional and modern treatment in Senegal (Diop & Ndiaye 2007).

In summary, action required to reduce the epilepsy treatment gap in Africa, and consequently mortality including sudden death, demands a multidisciplinary approach. The reduction of predictable causes of epilepsy, and better management of seizures, pregnancy, and child health, must be considered as priorities.

Amadou Gallo Diop
Professor of Neurology
Epileptology and Neurosciences, University of Dakar, Senegal.

South Africa

The Greek author and philosopher Plato wrote: *'Must not all things at the last be swallowed up in death? It is however, particularly tragic when death comes without warning, and claims a child or young adult not 'at the last' as opined by Plato, but in the prime of their lives. This has a great impact not only on society, but also on the medical personnel who are responsible for determining the cause of the sudden death'.* (Dempers & Van Vuuren 2006)

The psychological impact of sudden unexplained death in epilepsy (SUDEP) is probably the most difficult aspect in medical practice, especially within a country with diverse cultural beliefs and practices surrounding the cause and treatment of epilepsy. In South Africa, less attention has been paid to SUDEP. True sudden unexplained deaths in the country are viewed as "unnatural deaths'. However, people suffering from epilepsy are deemed to be at high risk of SUDEP (Dempers & Van Vuuren 2006).

From an African point of view, SUDEP or any unexplained death is hard to accept and comprehend by bereaved families. For most African communities, there must always be an answer to the following questions: *What is the cause of the persons' death? Why did he/she die suddenly? How did he/she die? When and where? Who is responsible for the death?*

These answers are needed prior to the burial of the deceased, to provide explanations to the family and close relatives about the progression of the person's illness, the treatment and care prior to death. This task is performed by a chosen family representative, who is usually referred to as a *'carer of the deceased person'*, and whose role is to address doubts, fears, suspicions, questions or concerns that the family or extended family may have regarding sudden death of a family member. For example, in some instances, where bewitchment is suspected to be the cause of the unnatural or sudden unexplained death, the suspected perpetrator may be ostracized. On the other hand, some families may consult with traditional healers to seek explanations for the cause of death in order to get closure. Others may accept sudden unexplained death as 'Gods Will'.

SUDEP may have great psychological impact on the family, especially as epilepsy is a condition that is clouded by superstitious beliefs and practices surrounding its cause and treatment. These cultural beliefs and practices vary among communities in the country (Eastman 2005).

SUDEP is not only a concern for society but also for the health care professionals (Dempers & Van Vuuren, 2006). With the poor understanding and management of epilepsy in the country (Keikelame & Swartz 2007), SUDEP becomes an issue of critical concern.

In 1998, I conducted a study in a peri-urban township in Cape Town. The study explored what parents of children with epilepsy understood as the cause and management of their children's condition. I found that parents used inappropriate first aid care for seizures, such as 'putting cloths or spoons in the mouth during a seizure or giving medication once seizures have stopped'. Another study in Limpopo province found that some people used 'smoke inhalations' to treat epilepsy (Mangena-Netshikweta 2003), perhaps in an effort to chase away evil spirits which they may deem to be the cause of the illness. These actions, in my view, could be risk factors for SUDEP. Therefore, collaborative research and promoting public awareness about SUDEP in the country is critical.

Mpoe Johannah Keikelame
Member, Epilepsy South Africa, Western Cape Branch, Cape Town.

Acknowledgements: Mr James Irlam, Ms Claudia Naidu and Ms Bonani Dube of the Primary Health Care Directorate, University of Cape Town.

Mexico

The mortality rate in México according to statistics recorded in 2010 is 4.86 per 1000 persons in a population of more than 106 million people. The main causes of death are degenerative chronic diseases, whereas transmissible diseases are being reported with diminishing frequency.

Searching for information about death certificates, we found that these documents are filled out heterogeneously and although there is an official guide for completing the forms there is still a lack of consistency in reporting. We tried to consult the record of certificates but the information is not available on the internet. We know that a great number of certificates register cardiac or respiratory arrest as the direct cause of death and although there are other spaces to add the underlying diseases which lead to the final and direct cause of death this information is not reported in the statistics available. One option to describe a cause of death is 'symptoms and signs not well defined'. Another is 'other causes'. These categories would include multiple diseases that perhaps are used to include epilepsy.

Speaking about mortality related to epilepsy, the available information in medical literature says that the life expectancy is similar to the general population. In theory differences could exist because people with epilepsy have a higher risk of accidents or fatal complications, but in Mexico we do not have reports about any differences.

In relation to deaths which might fit the SUDEP definition we do not have any reliable information. Mortality related to epilepsy is reported as being due to accidents, the consequence of seizures, or the consequence of status epilepticus. The reports of the deaths do not fit the concept of SUDEP.

Four years ago, we did a survey about accidents suffered by people with epilepsy who attended the monthly information sessions of the Mexican Chapter of the IBE. We found that 30% had suffered some kind of injury because of their seizures but almost none required hospitalization. On the other hand we know that 5 members of the group have died in the last ten years; one was a female hospitalized because of frequent seizures, one died in the street, and the others were not witnessed. None of the cases included an autopsy, so we do not have more information. It is possible that one or two could have had been a SUDEP death.

In our information sessions, booklets, and webpage we try to transmit optimism about living life with epilepsy and we reject stigmatization of epilepsy in the social environment. We know that the risk of SUDEP is greater in non-controlled epilepsy and an important topic in our information sessions is the risk of death related to seizures, as a consequence of fatal accidents or status epilepticus. We try always to encourage people to have good and constant antiepileptic treatment in order to diminish risks and improve their quality of life. Promoting awareness about the importance of good compliance to antiepileptic treatment in order to achieve the best control of epilepsy is not easy, so we discuss the physical risks and the possibility of intellectual damage. We speak about SUDEP only if somebody asks about the topic.

We have not carried out any surveys about SUDEP because of the current limitations which exist to demonstrate it as a cause of death. However, it would be interesting to gather information about death related to epilepsy with its multiple causes, including SUDEP.

This communication encourages us to design and realize a future survey in the countries of our Latin American region in order to find out the causes of death related to epilepsy. This information could be of high interest to prevent complications and death in our population with epilepsy.

Lilia Núñez-Orozco
President of Mexican Chapter and Latin American Committee of IBE.

France

Specialists in the field of epileptology in France know about the question of unexpected sudden death in people with epilepsy but this information is not readily available for the patients, their families, general physicians, or the public at large.

There are various explanations for this silence about SUDEP:

■ Social representations of people with epilepsy are generally negative and associated with the risk of accidents. This hampers information flow to various sectors including insurance, schooling, employment, regulations and rules. It also damages the quality of everyday life for people with epilepsy and affects the possibility of social inclusion.

■ Talking about SUDEP will increase existing anxieties which patients and their families may have towards seizures, especially tonic-clonic seizures, the loss of consciousness, possible serious injury and death and eventual serious accidents doesn't enlist a deeper concern.

■ Patients and their families don't ask to be kept informed about this risk (perhaps they are not aware that it is an issue).

Of those who have experienced SUDEP, many prefer not to speak about it, a minority blame their doctors and begin law suits for what they see as poor care or the lack of medical surveillance. A handful have formed groups that propose to support other grieving families.

Most importantly, many healthcare professionals hesitate to prepare their patients and families for the eventuality of a SUDEP because they themselves lack information.

Additional obstacles to SUDEP knowledge include the lack of in-depth epidemiological studies and the fact that death certificates are rarely documented and autopsies are unusual. Also the files of patients who have died from SUDEP are often unavailable. Where they are available they may be incomplete and unreliable.

Moreover, the criteria that identify SUDEP are not clearly defined, nor common to all the published studies. Do the SUDEP deaths have to be limited to inexplicable deaths occurring rapidly after a seizure, allowing one to surmise that the seizure is the unique cause of death because of the cardiac arrest, or can they be also related to other inexplicable causes happening well after seizures thus bringing into play other factors.

In our study (Beaussart-Defaye & Beaussart 2009) we analyzed seventy cases of unexplained deaths. We have followed these cases for years, so our data is complete and verified. Only 7.3% died rapidly or in a few hours time after a seizure and most often at home (75%). If the deaths were declared in the morning (52.5%), in patients who were alone and asleep, it was not always possible to confirm or rule out a nocturnal seizure that may or may not have occurred.

In our analysis we have stated, as in other published studies, that the highest risk is associated with epilepsies which are: cryptogenic with partial seizures and secondary generalizations (57.6%); drug-resistant (52.5%); or related to personal antecedents (40.7% of neonatal convulsions, meningitis, or cerebral motor infirmities). High risk is also associated with anxiety, depressive, intellectual (36.1%), or psychiatric (30.5%) disorders. We have also observed that SUDEP is more frequent in men than in women. Deaths occurred principally between the ages of 21 and 40 (50.8%) but also between the ages of 9 and 12 (2.9%) and after the age of 40 (35.6%).

The French League Against Epilepsy and the French Foundation for the Research on Epilepsies have recently set up an epidemiological network watch to survey mortality in epilepsy. In the end such collected data should locate the causes of death and demonstrate the differences between those which can be classified as SUDEP and those which stem from progressive syndromes with a fatal prognosis, from accidents ending in death, from suicides, or from status epilepticus

Currently, with new French laws concerning the organization of care, the implementation of medical and socio-medical assistance, and therapeutic education being developed, it would be useful to approach patients with epilepsy, and their families, to inform them about the risks of SUDEP.

This strategy will be facilitated by the eventual determination of risk factors according to the clinical and socio-psychological profiles of the patients, so that preventive strategies can be suggested.

Interdisciplinary programs of research permitting a mutual sharing of results from different countries would be very useful to implement this new program.

Jacqueline Beaussart-Defaye
Executive Director, AISPACE, France.

Brazil

Sudden unexpected death in epilepsy (SUDEP) remains an extremely serious and common event. Epidemiological studies indicate that SUDEP is responsible for 7.5% to 17% of all deaths in epilepsy and has an incidence among adults between 1:500 and 1:1,000 patient-years. Furthermore, several risk factors (refractoriness of the epileptic condition, presence of generalized tonic-clonic seizures, polytherapy with antiepileptic drugs, young age, duration of the seizure disorder, early onset of epilepsy, winter temperatures) and different mechanisms (respiratory and cardiovascular) are already well defined for SUDEP.

Although neglected in earlier literature, the last 15 years have witnessed an increase in scientific research on SUDEP. However, it is important to emphasize that most of these studies were conducted in adults and, unfortunately, we still have little data regarding SUDEP in children. In the last year our research group in Brazil reviewed the occurrence of SUDEP in children in our epilepsy unit over an 8-year period. Our study evaluated the incidence of SUDEP in a cohort of children aged between zero and 18 years, evaluated in the Clinical Hospital of Ribeirão Preto in 2000 and followed until June 2008.

Briefly, from 835 patients evaluated 12 had suffered SUDEP and nearly all of the SUDEP cases in our children were related to chronic uncontrolled epilepsy (seizures; daily--50.0%, two to four/week--41.7%, monthly--8.3%). Furthermore, the presence of generalized tonic-clonic seizures and polytherapy with antiepileptic drugs were also highlighted as risk factors in our study. It is interesting to note that the results of our study agree with previous studies in children and adults with epilepsy, where increased mortality was recorded in those individuals who had not responded to treatment.

After these results, some suggestions should be highlighted: 1 – SUDEP in children is not a rare event; 2 – improved seizure control by treatment (pharmacological or surgical) seems to be one of the most important measures to prevent SUDEP in our children; 3 – some preventive strategies against SUDEP, already proposed and well accepted among epileptologists, might also have great value if adopted for our children with epilepsy. These measures include reduction of stress, participation in physical activity and sports (under supervision of a qualified professional), dietary management (e.g., omega-3 supplementation), supervision at night, and family members' knowledge of cardiopulmonary resuscitation (CPR) and defibrillator use; 4 –The American Epilepsy Society and the Epilepsy Foundation Joint Task Force for SUDEP has promoted multidisciplinary investigation to identify additional areas of research for mechanisms underlying SUDEP. It would be interesting to extend this action directly to the pediatric neurology field, i.e., evaluate and establish new strategies (research directions, social, cultural and educational efforts) related to the phenomenon of SUDEP in children.

Overall, SUDEP in children is a 'new' scientific area for research and we could make great strides. For that, we must do this cooperatively and cross-nationally as this is truly an international issue.

Fulvio A. Scorza, Vera C. Terra, Ricardo M. Arida & Esper A. Cavalheiro
Disciplina de Neurologia Experimental. Universidade Federal de São Paulo/Escola Paulista de Medicina. (UNIFESP/EPM). São Paulo, Brasil.

Canada

Early in 2008 pediatric neurologist Dr Elizabeth Donner and I started SUDEP Aware, a non-profit organization dedicated to promoting knowledge and understanding of sudden unexpected death in epilepsy (SUDEP) through education, research and support.

For Dr Donner, who had previously conducted a 10-year review of paediatric SUDEP in Ontario, this was an opportunity to further her involvement in, and contribution towards, a field that has intrigued her and one she firmly feels needs advancement.

For me, having lost a sister to SUDEP in 2007 and been unable to find any information or support in North America, this seemed the only option towards helping to address the issue and trying to prevent others from going through such a devastating experience.

The past four years have seen a similar reaction in other families impacted by SUDEP. In the US, half a dozen foundations have been set up to help improve awareness of SUDEP and to raise funds for epilepsy support. In Canada, one such organization, the Caroline Cunningham Foundation for Epilepsy was established in 2009 and works to raise funds for research, kid's summer camp support and seizure-response dog sponsorship. In many cases, foundations have established working partnerships with their local epilepsy organizations in order to help them achieve their goals. This has increased the profile of SUDEP with the epilepsy organizations and has reinforced the strong need for them to provide SUDEP-specific information and support to their members. A significant rise in the number of fundraising events, held in memory of a loved one lost to SUDEP, is now evident. In Canada, with the support of the Canadian Epilepsy Alliance (CEA) and others, awareness is starting to spread.

There is still, however, a very long way to go. Here, as elsewhere, the actual incidence of SUDEP has not yet been comprehensively determined. Dr Donner has been awarded a grant from CURE to implement the first registry of SUDEP deaths in children, with the significant objective of determining those children at greatest risk of SUDEP and to ascertain possible protective measures. Of course, this work relies very heavily on the accurate identification of deaths attributable to SUDEP; the appropriate recording of the deaths and the terminology used. It also requires individual cases to be logged with the relevant researchers for the accurate collation of data.

To this end, SUDEP Aware is actively working to promote communication between families, death investigators, medical professionals and researchers, to ensure timely and appropriate information exchange.

SUDEP Aware also assists researchers in the procurement of blood and tissue samples. These are used to investigate genetic risk factors that may predispose an individual to epilepsy and to sudden death. To date, Baylor College of Medicine has identified two genes that may explain certain SUDEP cases. By participating in such studies, families can take some small comfort from the knowledge that sharing information will assist researchers in their quest to identify the etiology of SUDEP.

The prevalent cause of frustration and complaint from most SUDEP-bereaved families is the fact that they were not informed about the risks of SUDEP prior to the loss of their loved one. Unfortunately, this situation remains an issue even today. SUDEP Aware strongly believes that knowledge is the necessary catalyst for prevention and has been working with like-minded organizations to develop a strategy to increase awareness of SUDEP.

Through ongoing collaboration and the assistance of the epilepsy support community, a campaign to heighten awareness throughout the professional and lay communities of North America and beyond is under way. It is a multi-dimensional, sustained effort to champion the need for more medical research; mobilize and share resources (such as educational material, discussion tools and support) from healthcare, academic and advocacy groups; encourage increased discussion and promotion of SUDEP knowledge; and generate action from professionals and the general public in support of the campaign.

Increasing awareness of SUDEP is the first critical step on the road to improving understanding of this devastating outcome of epilepsy. From awareness comes improved identification of cases, and from research emerges knowledge and the increased likelihood of finding the cause and/or methods of prevention of SUDEP.

Tamzin Jeffs

Glossary

A Level. Advanced Level General Certificate of Education, part of the tertiary further education system [UK].

Absence Seizure. A non-convulsive generalized seizure marked by the abrupt, transient loss or impairment of consciousness (usually a blank stare, not subsequently remembered).

Adenosine. A chemical important to human function.

AED. Antiepileptic Drugs, used to treat seizures in epilepsy.

AES. American Epilepsy Society www.aesnet.org [USA].

AIDS. Acquired Immune Deficiency Syndrome, a disease involving a severe loss of the body's cellular immunity, which greatly lowers its resistance to infection and malignancy.

Apnea. The temporary cessation of breathing.

Arrhythmia. A disorder of heart rate or rhythm.

Aspiration. The sucking in of fluid or foreign matter into the airway when drawing breath.

Asystole. A state in which the heart ceases to beat.

Autonomic. Pertaining to the autonomic nervous system which is the portion of the nervous system that is responsible for the unconscious regulation of vital bodily functions such as breathing and digestion.

Autopsy. See *post mortem.*

Beta blockers. A type of drug that blocks the action of the *sympathetic nervous system* of the heart, resulting in a relief of stress on the heart.

Bradycardia. The slowing down of the heart rate.

Capnography. The monitoring of the concentration or partial pressure of carbon dioxide (CO_2) in the respiratory gases.

Cardiac repolarization. The phase of the cardiac cycle during which the electrical excitation of the heart muscle returns to the resting condition.

Cardio. Of, or relating to, the heart.

CDC. Centers for Disease Control and Prevention www.cdc.gov [USA].

CEA. Canadian Epilepsy Alliance www.epilepsymatters.com [Canada].

Channelopathy disease. Caused by disturbed function of ion channels or the proteins that regulate them.

CO_2. Carbon Dioxide.

Combination Therapy. See *polytherapy.*

Complex partial seizure. An epileptic seizure that originates in a specific area (focus) of the brain associated with impairment of consciousness.

CT scan. Computerized Axial Tomography or CAT scan, a sectional view of the body constructed by x-ray computed tomography.

CURE. Citizens United in Research for Epilepsy www.cureepilepsy.org [USA].

DBA/2 mice. Dilute Brown Non-Agouti mice (refers to coat colour).

Defibrillator. An electronic device used to restore rhythm of a fibrillating heart by applying an electric shock to it.

DNA. Deoxyribonucleic Acid.

Dravet's syndrome. Also known as Severe Myoclonic Epilepsy of Infancy (SMEI); a rare and catastrophic form of epilepsy for which there is currently no cure.

ECG. Electrocardiogram, records changes in electrical potential during the heartbeat.

Edema. Abnormal excess accumulation of fluid in the cavities or tissues of the body.

EEG. Electroencephalogram, a diagnostic test of brain electrical activity.

EF. Epilepsy Foundation www.efa.org [USA].

EKG. See ECG

Electrocerebral. Pertaining to electrical activity in the brain.

EMU. Epilepsy monitoring unit.

Epilepsy. A neurological condition characterized by two or more unprovoked seizures.

ER. Emergency Room.

Fibrillation. Muscular twitching involving individual muscle fibres acting without coordination.

GP, General Practitioner. Family doctor.

GPRD. General Practice Research Database [UK].

GPS. Global Positioning System.

Grand mal seizures. See *tonic-clonic seizures.*

HRV. Heart Rate Variability.

Hypercapnia. Presence of excess carbon dioxide in the blood.

Hypoventilation. Deficient ventilation of the lungs resulting in decreased levels of oxygen and/or increase levels of carbon dioxide content in the blood.

Hypoxemia. Deficient oxygenation of the blood.

Hypoxia. Deficiency of oxygen reaching the tissues of the body.

IBE. International Bureau for Epilepsy www.ibe-epilepsy.org.

ICD-10. International Classification of Diseases, 10th and most recent revision.

Ictal. Relating to a seizure.

Idiopathic Epilepsy. Epilepsy arising spontaneously or from an unknown cause.

ILAE. International League Against Epilepsy www.ilae-epilepsy.org.

Intractable Epilepsy. Epilepsy that is not easily managed or controlled.

Ion channel. A structure in the membrane of nerve and muscle cells through which ions enter and exit the cell. In an epileptic seizure, the ion channels of the neurons of the brain are affected, so that there is a much greater outflow of ions than normal.

KCNA1 gene. Or, potassium voltage-gated channel (KCN), shaker-related subfamily, member 1 gene. It provides instructions for making one part (the alpha subunit) of a potassium channel called Kv1.1.

KCNH2 gene. Or, potassium voltage-gated channel (KCN), subfamily H, member 2 gene. It provides instructions for making potassium channels in heart muscle, which play a major role in maintaining regular heart rhythm.

KCNQ1 gene. Or, potassium voltage-gated channel (KCN), KQT-like subfamily, member 1 gene. It provides instructions for making potassium channels in heart muscle which play a major role in maintaining regular heart rhythm.

LQTS, Long QT Syndrome. A disorder of the heart's electrical activity.

Mortemus. MORTality in Epilepsy Monitoring Unit Study [France].

MRI. Magnetic Resonance Imaging.

Neurodeficit. Neurological deficit, any defect or absence of function of a peripheral nerve or a system.

Neuron. A nerve cell.

NGO. Non government organization.

NIH. National Institutes of Health www.nih.gov [USA]

NINDS. National Institute of Neurological Disorders and Stroke www.ninds.nih.gov [USA]

NREM. Non Rapid Eye Movement.

Oxygen saturation/desaturation. A measure of how much oxygen the blood is carrying as a percentage of the maximum it could carry (saturation); when the blood does not have enough oxygen (desaturation).

Parasympathetic nervous system. The part of the autonomic nervous system responsible for decreasing blood pressure, slowing heart rate and increasing digestion.

Petit Mal. See *absence seizures.*

PGES. Postictal Generalized Electroencephalographic Suppression.

Placebo. An inert or innocuous substance.

Polytherapy. The use of more than one drug.

Postictal. Relating to the period following a seizure.

Post mortem. Or autopsy, is the examination of a dead body to determine cause of death.

Prodrome. Early symptom indicating the onset of a disease or illness.

PUFA. Polyunsaturated Fatty Acids.

Pulse Oximetry. A non-invasive method of monitoring the level of oxygen in blood.

QT Interval. A time interval on an electrocardiogram (ECG/EKG) that represents the beginning of the heart ventricles' contraction until the end of relaxation.

REM. Rapid Eye Movement.

SCN5A gene. Or, sodium channel (SCN), voltage-gated, type V, alpha subunit gene. It provides instructions for making sodium channels, which are abundant in heart muscle and play a major role in maintaining normal heart rhythm.

Serotonin. Also called 5-HT or 5-hydroxytryptamine, a neurotransmitter (substance used to transmit nerve impulses across synapses) and powerful vasoconstrictor.

SIDS. Sudden Infant Death Syndrome.

SIGN. Scottish Intercollegiate Guideline Network, develops evidence based clinical practice guidelines for the National Health Service in Scotland www.sign.ac.uk [UK].

SMR. Standardized Mortality Rate.

SSRI. Serotonin Reuptake Inhibitor, class of antidepressants that inhibit the inactivation of the neurotransmitter serotonin by blocking its reuptake by nerve cell endings.

Status Epilepticus. A single prolonged seizure or a series of seizures without intervening full recovery of consciousness.

SUDEP Research Initiative. A research collaboration between King's College, London and Epilepsy Bereaved [UK].

Sympathetic nervous system. The part of the autonomic nervous system responsible for 'fight or flight' response: increased heart rate, raising blood pressure, decreasing digestion; opposite to *parasympathetic nervous system.*

Symptomatic Epilepsy. Epilepsy arising from a particular cause (eg brain damage).

Syncope. Or fainting, temporary loss of consciousness resulting from insufficient blood flow to the brain.

Tachyarrhythmia. Rapid irregular heartbeat.

Tachycardia. Speeding up of the heart rate.

Terminal Remission. Refers to patients still in remission (no seizures for 5 or more years) at the end of a follow-up period.

Tonic-clonic seizures. Generalized seizures associated with loss of consciousness that begin with the body stiffening (tonic phase) followed by rhythmic jerking (clonic phase).

Toxicology. A branch of science concerned with poisons, their nature, effects, and detection.

UCL. University College London [UK].

Vagus nerve. The tenth cranial nerve and part of the autonomic nervous system.

Vagus nerve stimulation (VNS). A procedure involving external stimulation of the vagus nerve which can lead to an improvement of some forms of epilepsy.

Verbal Autopsy. Is a method of ascertaining cause of death from the collection of information regarding symptoms, signs and circumstances preceding death obtained from the deceased's caretakers and witnesses present.

WHO. World Health Organization www.who.int

Bibliography

Aldenkamp, AP, Overweg, J, Gutter, T, Beun, AM, Diepman, L & Mulder, OG 1996, 'Effect of epilepsy, seizures and epileptiform EEG discharges on cognitive function', *Acta Neurol Scand*, vol. 93, no. 4, pp. 253-9.

Annegers, JF 1997, 'United States perspective on definitions and classifications', *Epilepsia*, vol. 38, Suppl 11, pp. S9-12.

Annegers, JF & Coan, SP 1999, 'SUDEP: overview of definitions and review of incidence data', *Seizure*, vol. 8, no. 6, pp. 347-52.

Annegers, JF, Coan, SP, Hauser, WA & Leestma, J 2000, 'Epilepsy, vagal nerve stimulation by the NCP system, all-cause mortality, and sudden, unexpected, unexplained death', *Epilepsia*, vol. 41, no. 5, pp. 549-53.

Annegers, JF, Hauser, WA & Shirts, SB 1984, 'Heart disease mortality and morbidity in patients with epilepsy', *Epilepsia*, vol. 25, no. 6, pp. 699-704.

Babloyantz, A & Destexhe, A 1986, 'Low-dimensional chaos in an instance of epilepsy', *Proc Natl Acad Sci* USA, vol. 83, no. 10, pp. 3513-7.

Badawy, R, Macdonell, R, Jackson, G & Berkovic, S 2009, 'The peri-ictal state: cortical excitability changes within 24 h of a seizure', *Brain*, vol. 132, Pt 4, pp. 1013-21.

Bagdy, G, Kecskemeti, V, Riba, P & Jakus, R 2007, 'Serotonin and epilepsy', *J Neurochem*, vol. 100, no. 4, pp. 857-73.

Banerjee, TK, Ray, BK, Das, SK, Hazra, A, Ghosal, MK, Chaudhuri, A, Roy, T & Raut, DK 2010, 'A longitudinal study of epilepsy in Kolkata, India', *Epilepsia*, vol. 51, no. 12, pp. 2384-91.

Bateman, LM, Li, CS, Lin, TC & Seyal, M 2010, 'Serotonin reuptake inhibitors are associated with reduced severity of ictal hypoxemia in medically refractory partial epilepsy', *Epilepsia*, vol. 51, no. 10, pp. 2211-14.

Bateman, LM, Li, CS & Seyal, M 2008, 'Ictal hypoxemia in localization-related epilepsy: analysis of incidence, severity and risk factors', *Brain*, vol. 131, Pt 12, pp. 3239-45.

Bateman, LM, Spitz, M & Seyal, M 2010, 'Ictal hypoventilation contributes to cardiac arrhythmia and SUDEP: report on two deaths in video-EEG-monitored patients', *Epilepsia*, vol. 51, no. 5, pp. 916-20.

Beaussart-Defaye, J & Beaussart, M 2009, *Soigner les epilepsies: comprendre les maladies, accompagner les malades*, Elsevier-Masson, Issy-les-Moulineaux.

Bell, GS, Sinha, S, Tisi, J, Stephani, C, Scott, CA, Harkness, WF, McEvoy, AW, Peacock, JL, Walker, MC, Smith, SJ, Duncan, JS & Sander, JW 2010, 'Premature mortality in refractory partial epilepsy: does surgical treatment make a difference?', *J Neurol Neurosurg Psychiatry*, vol. 81, no. 7, pp. 716-8.

Berg, AT, Shinnar, S, Testa, FM, Levy, SR, Smith, SN & Beckerman, B 2004, 'Mortality in childhood-onset epilepsy', *Arch Pediatr Adolesc Med*, vol. 158, no. 12, pp. 1147-52.

Brodie, MJ & Holmes, GL 2008, 'Should all patients be told about sudden unexpected death in epilepsy (SUDEP)? Pros and Cons', *Epilepsia*, vol. 49, Suppl 9, pp. 99-101.

Brundtland, GH 2002, 'Welcome: The WHO view and launch of the second phase of the Global Campaign Against Epilepsy', Epilepsia, vol. 43 Suppl 6, pp. 5-6.

Buchanan, GF & Richerson, GB 2010, 'Central serotonin neurons are required for arousal to CO2', Proc Natl Acad Sci USA, vol. 107, no. 37, pp. 16354-9.

Camfield, CS, Camfield, PR & Veugelers, PJ 2002, 'Death in children with epilepsy: a population-based study', Lancet, vol. 359, no. 9321, pp. 1891-5.

Camfield, P & Camfield, C 2005, 'Sudden unexpected death in people with epilepsy: a pediatric perspective', Semin Pediatr Neurol, vol. 12, no. 1, pp. 10-4.

Carpio, A, Bharucha, NE, Jallon, P, Beghi, E, Campostrini, R, Zorzetto, S & Mounkoro, PP 2005, 'Mortality of epilepsy in developing countries', Epilepsia, vol. 46, Suppl 11, pp. 28-32.

Casdagli, MC, Lasemidis, LD, Savit, RS, Gilmore, RL, Roper, SN & Sackellares, JC 1997, 'Non-linearity in invasive EEG recordings from patients with temporal lobe epilepsy', Electroencephalogr Clin Neurophysiol, vol. 102, no. 2, pp. 98-105.

Chen, RC, Chang, YC, Chen, TH, Wu, HM & Liou, HH 2005, 'Mortality in adult patients with epilepsy in Taiwan', Epileptic Disord, vol. 7, no. 3, pp. 213-9.

Cramer, JA, Glassman, M & Rienzi, V 2002, 'The relationship between poor medication compliance and seizures', Epilepsy Behav, vol. 3, no. 4, pp. 338-42.

Davis, KA, Sturges, BK, Vite, CH, Ruedebusch, V, Worrell, G, Gardner, AB, Leyde, K, Sheffield, WD & Litt, B 2011, 'A novel implanted device to wirelessly record and analyze continuous intracranial canine EEG', Epilepsy Res, June 13 [Epub ahead of print].

Davis, KL, Candrilli, SD & Edin, HM 2007, 'Prevalence and cost impact of nonadherence with antiepilepsy drugs among adults in a managed care population', paper presented to Academy of Managed Care Pharmacy (AMCP)19th Annual Meeting Showcase, San Diego, CA.

Day, SM, Wu, YW, Strauss, DJ, Shavelle, RM & Reynolds, RJ 2005, 'Causes of death in remote symptomatic epilepsy', Neurology, vol. 65, no. 2, pp. 216-22.

Decoufle, P & Autry, A 2002, 'Increased mortality in children and adolescents with developmental disabilities', Paediatr Perinat Epidemiol, vol. 16, no. 4, pp. 375-82.

Delogu, AB, Spinelli, A, Battaglia, D, Dravet, C, De Nisco, A, Saracino, A, Romagnoli, C, Lanza, GA & Crea, F 2011, 'Electrical and autonomic cardiac function in patients with Dravet syndrome', Epilepsia, vol. 52 Suppl 2, pp. 55-8.

Dempers, J & Van Vuuren, RJ 2006, 'Sudden Unexplained death in adults - an approach', CMWE, vol. 24, no. 3, pp. 116-9.

Ding, D, Wang, W, Wu, J, Ma, G, Dai, X, Yang, B, Wang, T, Yuan, C, Hong, Z, de Boer, HM, Prilipko, L & Sander, JW 2006, 'Premature mortality in people with epilepsy in rural China: a prospective study', Lancet Neurol, vol. 5, no. 10, pp. 823-7.

Diop, AG, Hesdorffer, DC, Logroscino, G & Hauser, WA 2005, 'Epilepsy and mortality in Africa: a review of the literature', Epilepsia, vol. 46 no. Supp 11, pp. 33-5.

Diop, AG, Mandlhate, C, Zenebe, GD, Grunitzky, EK, Kalangu, KN, Matuja, W, Pahl, K, Mielke, J, Meinardi, H, Prilipko, L, de Boer, H & Agoussou, T (eds) 2004, *Epilepsy in the African region: bridging the gap (AFR/ MNH/04.1)*, World Health Organization.

Diop, AG & Ndiaye, IP 2007, 'Organization of epilepsy healthcare in Senegal', in P Engel & T Pedley (eds), *Epilepsy: a comprehensive textbook*, 2nd edn, Lippincott, Williams & Wilkins.

Diop, AG, Sene-Diouf, F, Preux, PM & Ndiaye, IP 2003, 'Prognosis of epilepsy in Africa', in P Jallon, A Berg, O Dulac & WA Hauser (eds), *Prognosis of epilepsies*, John Libbey Eurotext, Paris, pp. 135-46.

Doheny, K 2011, Precautions cut sudden death risk of epilepsy, viewed July 9 2011, <http://www.webmd.com/epilepsy/news/20110705/precautions-cut-sudden-death-risk-of-epilepsy>.

Donner, EJ, Smith, CR & Snead, OC, 3rd 2001, 'Sudden unexplained death in children with epilepsy', *Neurology*, vol. 57, no. 3, pp. 430-4.

Duncan, JS, Sander, JW, Sisodiya, SM & Walker, MC 2006, 'Adult epilepsy', *Lancet*, vol. 367, no. 9516, pp. 1087-100.

Eastman, R 2005, 'Epilepsy in South Africa', *Acta Neurol Scand Suppl*, vol. 181, pp. 8-11.

Elliot, WJ 2001, 'Cyclic and circadian variations in cardiovascular events', *Am J Hypertens*, vol. 14, no. 9 Pt 2, pp. 291S-5S.

'Epilepsy must become a higher priority in Europe', 2010, *The Lancet Neurology*, no. 10, p. 941, viewed July 17 2011, DOI doi:10.1016/S1474-4422(10)70226-X, <http://www.thelancet.com/journals/laneur/article/PIIS1474-4422(10)70226-X/fulltext?version =printerFriendly>.

Faught, E, Duh, MS, Weiner, JR, Guerin, A & Cunnington, MC 2008, 'Nonadherence to antiepileptic drugs and increased mortality: findings from the RANSOM Study', *Neurology*, vol. 71, no. 20, pp. 1572-8.

Faught, RE, Weiner, JR, Guerin, A, Cunnington, MC & Duh, MS 2009, 'Impact of nonadherence to antiepileptic drugs on health care utilization and costs: findings from the RANSOM study', *Epilepsia*, vol. 50, no. 3, pp. 501-9.

Ficker, DM, So, EL, Shen, WK, Annegers, JF, O'Brien, PC, Cascino, GD & Belau, PG 1998, 'Population-based study of the incidence of sudden unexplained death in epilepsy', *Neurology*, vol. 51, no. 5, pp. 1270-4.

Finsterer, J & Stollberger, C 2011, 'Cardiac and pulmonary risk factors and pathomechanisms of sudden unexplained death in epilepsy patients', in CM Lathers, PL Schraeder, MW Bungo & J Leestma (eds), *Sudden death in epilepsy: forensic and clinical issues*, CRC Press, Boca Raton, pp. 679-92.

Fischhoff, B 1999, 'What do patients want? help in making effective choices', *Eff Clinc Pract*, vol. 2, no. 4, pp. 198-200.

Forsgren, L, Edvinsson, SO, Nystrom, L & Blomquist, HK 1996, 'Influence of epilepsy on mortality in mental retardation: an epidemiologic study', *Epilepsia*, vol. 37, no. 10, pp. 956-63.

Forsgren, L, Hauser, WA, Olafsson, E, Sander, JW, Sillanpaa, M & Tomson, T 2005, 'Mortality of epilepsy in developed countries: a review', *Epilepsia*, vol. 46 Suppl 11, pp. 18-27.

Fukuda, M, Suzuki, Y, Hino, H, Morimoto, T & Ishii, E 2011, 'Activation of central adenosine A(2A) receptors lowers the seizure threshold of hyperthermia-induced seizure in childhood rats', *Seizure*, vol. 20, no. 2, pp. 156-9.

Geerts, A, Arts, WF, Stroink, H, Peeters, E, Brouwer, O, Peters, B, Laan, L & van Donselaar, C 2010, 'Course and outcome of childhood epilepsy: a 15-year follow-up of the Dutch Study of Epilepsy in Childhood', *Epilepsia*, vol. 51, no. 7, pp. 1189-97.

Glasscock, E, Yoo, JW, Chen, TT, Klassen, TL & Noebels, JL 2010, 'Kv1.1 potassium channel deficiency reveals brain-driven cardiac dysfunction as a candidate mechanism for sudden unexplained death in epilepsy', *J Neurosci*, vol. 30, no. 15, pp. 5167-75.

Goldman, AM, Glasscock, E, Yoo, J, Chen, TT, Klassen, TL & Noebels, JL 2009, 'Arrhythmia in heart and brain: KCNQ1 mutations link epilepsy and sudden unexplained death', *Sci Transl Med*, vol. 1, no. 2, p. 2ra6.

Hancox, JC & Witchel, HJ 2000, 'Psychotropic drugs, HERG, and the heart', *Lancet*, vol. 356, no. 9227, p. 428.

Hanna, J & Panelli, R 2011, 'Challenges in overcoming ethical, legal and communication barriers in SUDEP', in CM Lathers, PL Schraeder, MW Bungo & JE Leestma (eds), *Sudden death in epilepsy: forensic and clinical issues*, CRC Press, Bosa Roca, pp. 915-35.

Hanna, NJ, Black, M, Sander, JWS, Smithson, WH, Appleton, R, Brown, S & Fish, DR 2002, *The national sentinel clinical audit of epilepsy related death: epilepsy - death in the shadows*, The Stationary Office.

Harnod, T, Yang, CC, Hsin, YL, Wang, PJ, Shieh, KR & Kuo, TB 2009, 'Heart rate variability in patients with frontal lobe epilepsy', *Seizure*, vol. 18, no. 1, pp. 21-5.

Hauser, WA, Annegers, JF & Elveback, LR 1980, 'Mortality in patients with epilepsy', *Epilepsia*, vol. 21, no. 4, pp. 399-412.

Herreros, B 2011, 'Cardiac channelopathies and sudden death', in CM Lathers, P Schraeder, MW Bungo & J Leestma (eds), *Sudden death in epilepsy: forensic and clinical issues*, CRC Press, Boca Raton, pp. 285-302.

Hesdorffer, DC, Tomson, T, Benn, E, Sander, JW, Nilsson, L, Langan, Y, Walczak, TS, Beghi, E, Brodie, MJ, Hauser, A, for the ILAE Commission on Epidemiology & Subcommission on Mortality 2011, 'Combined analysis of risk factors for SUDEP', *Epilepsia*, vol. 52, no. 6, pp. 1150-9.

Hirsch, LJ, Donner, EJ, So, EL, Jacobs, M, Nashef, L, Noebels, JL & Buchhalter, JR 2011, 'Abbreviated report of the NIH/NINDS workshop on sudden unexpected death in epilepsy', *Neurology*, vol. 76, no. 22, pp. 1932-8.

Hodges, MR, Tattersall, GJ, Harris, MB, McEvoy, SD, Richerson, DN, Deneris, ES, Johnson, RL, Chen, ZF & Richerson, GB 2008, 'Defects in breathing and thermoregulation in mice with near-complete absence of central serotonin neurons', *J Neurosci*, vol. 28, no. 10, pp. 2495-505.

Hotta, H, Koizumi, K & Stewart, M 2009, 'Cardiac sympathetic nerve activity during kainic acid-induced limbic cortical seizures in rats', *Epilepsia*, vol. 50, no. 4, pp. 923-7.

Hotta, H, Lazar, J, Orman, R, Koizumi, K, Shiba, K, Kamran, H & Stewart, M 2009, 'Vagus nerve stimulation-induced bradyarrhythmias in rats', *Auton Neurosci*, vol. 151, no. 2, pp. 98-105.

Hughes, JR 2009, 'A review of sudden unexpected death in epilepsy: prediction of patients at risk', *Epilepsy Behav*, vol. 14, no. 2, pp. 280-7.

Jallon, P 1997, 'Epilepsy in developing countries', *Epilepsia*, vol. 38, no. 10, pp. 1143-51.

Jehi, L 2010, 'Sudden death in epilepsy, surgery, and seizure outcomes: the interface between heart and brain', *Cleve Clin J Med*, vol. 77 Suppl 3, pp. S51-5.

Jilek-Aall, L & Rwiza, HT 1992, 'Prognosis of epilepsy in a rural African community: a 30-year follow-up of 164 patients in an outpatient clinic in rural Tanzania', *Epilepsia*, vol. 33, no. 4, pp. 645-50.

Johnson-Laird, PN 19893, *Mental models: towards a cognitive science of language, interference and consciousness*, Cambridge University Press, Cambridge

Johnson, JN, Hofman, N, Haglund, CM, Cascino, GD, Wilde, AA & Ackerman, MJ 2009, 'Identification of a possible pathogenic link between congenital long QT syndrome and epilepsy', *Neurology*, vol. 72, no. 3, pp. 224-31.

Kale, R 1997, 'Bringing epilepsy out of the shadows', BMJ, vol. 315, no. 7099, pp. 2-3.

Kalitzin, S, Parra, J, Velis, DN & Lopes da Silva, FH 2002, 'Enhancement of phase clustering in the EEG/MEG gamma frequency band anticipates transitions to paroxysmal epileptiform activity in epileptic patients with known visual sensitivity', *IEEE Trans Biomed Eng*, vol. 49, no. 11, pp. 1279-86.

Kanner, AM 2009, 'Depression and epilepsy: a review of multiple facets of their close relation', *Neurol Clin*, vol. 27, no. 4, pp. 865-80.

Keikelame, MJ & Swartz, L 2007, 'Parents' understanding of the causes and management of their children's epilepsy in Khjayelitsha, Cape Town', *South African Journal of Psychology*, vol. 37, pp. 307-15.

Kennelly, C & Riesel, J 2002, *Sudden death and epilepsy - the views and experiences of bereaved relatives and carers*, Epilepsy Bereaved.

Kinney, HC, Richerson, GB, Dymecki, SM, Darnall, RA & Nattie, EE 2009, 'The brainstem and serotonin in the sudden infant death syndrome', *Annu Rev Pathol*, vol. 4, pp. 517-50.

Koehler, SA, Schraeder, PL, Lathers, CM & Wecht, CH 2011, 'One-year postmortem forensic analysis of deaths in person with epilepsy', in CM Lathers, P Schraeder, MW

Bungo & J Leestma (eds), *Sudden death in epilepsy: forensic and clinical issues*, CRC Press, Boca Raton, pp. 145-58.

Kwan, P & Brodie, MJ 2007, 'Emerging drugs for epilepsy', *Expert Opin Emerg Drugs*, vol. 12, no. 3, pp. 407-22.

Lai, YC, Harrison, MA, Frei, MG & Osorio, I 2003, 'Inability of Lyapunov exponents to predict epileptic seizures', *Phys Rev Lett*, vol. 91, no. 6, p. 068102.

Lai, YC, Harrison, MA, Frei, MG & Osorio, I 2004, 'Controlled test for predictive power of Lyapunov exponents: their inability to predict epileptic seizures', *Chaos*, vol. 14, no. 3, pp. 630-42.

Langan, Y, Nashef, L & Sander, JW 2005, 'Case-control study of SUDEP', *Neurology*, vol. 64, no. 7, pp. 1131-3.

Lathers, CM 2009, 'Epilepsy and sudden death: personal reflections and call for global action', *Epilepsy Behav*, vol. 15, no. 3, pp. 269-77.

Lathers, CM 2011, 'Could beta blocker antiarrythmic and antiseizure activity help prevent SUDEP?', in CM Lathers, P Schraeder, MW Bungo & J Leestma (eds), *Sudden death in epilepsy: forensic and clinical issues*, CRC Press, Boca Raton, pp. 877-86.

Lathers, CM, Koehler, SA, Wecht, CH & Schraeder, PL 2003, 'Forensic antiepileptic drug levels in 2001 autopsy cases of sudden unexpected deaths in persons with epilepsy in Allegheny county Pennsylvania', paper presented to FDA science forum, Washington, DC.

Lathers, CM & Schraeder, P (eds) 1990, *Epilepsy and sudden death*, Marcel Dekker Inc, New York.

Lathers, CM & Schraeder, PL 2002, 'Clinical pharmacology: drugs as a benefit and/or risk in sudden unexpected death in epilepsy?', *J Clin Pharmacol*, vol. 42, no. 2, pp. 123-36.

Lathers, CM & Schraeder, PL 2006, 'Stress and sudden death', *Epilepsy Behav*, vol. 9, no. 2, pp. 236-42.

Lathers, CM & Schraeder, PL 2009, 'Verbal autopsies and SUDEP', *Epilepsy Behav*, vol. 14, no. 4, pp. 573-6.

Lathers, CM & Schraeder, P 2011a, 'Animal models for sudden unexpected death in persons with epilepsy', in CM Lathers, P Schraeder, MW Bungo & J Leestma (eds), *Sudden death in epilepsy: forensic and clinical issues*, CRC Press, Boca Raton, pp. 437-63.

Lathers, CM & Schraeder, PL 2011b, 'Clinical pharmacology and SUDEP', in CM Lathers, P Schraeder, MW Bungo & J Leestma (eds), *Sudden unexpected death in epilepsy: forensic and clinical issues*, CRC Press, Boca Raton, pp. 789-99.

Lathers, CM, Schraeder, PL & Bungo, MW 2008, 'The mystery of sudden death: mechanisms for risks', *Epilepsy Behav*, vol. 12, no. 1, pp. 3-24.

Lathers, CM, Schraeder, PL & Bungo, MW 2011, 'Neurocardiologic mechanistic risk factors in SUDEP', in CM Lathers, P Schraeder, MW Bungo & J Leestma (eds), *Sudden unexpected death in epilepsy: forensic and clinical issues*, CRC Press, Boca Raton, pp. 3-35.

Lathers, CM, Schraeder, PL & Claycamp, HG 2003, 'Clinical pharmacology of topiramate versus lamotrigine versus phenobarbital: comparison of efficacy and side effects using odds ratios', *J Clin Pharmacol*, vol. 43, no. 5, pp. 491-503.

Le Van Quyen, M, Martinerie, J, Baulac, M & Varela, F 1999, 'Anticipating epileptic seizures in real time by a non-linear analysis of similarity between EEG recordings', *Neuroreport*, vol. 10, no. 10, pp. 2149-55.

Leestma, JE 2011, 'Forensic considerations and sudden unexpected death in epilepsy', in CM Lathers, P Schraeder, MW Bungo & J Leestma (eds), *Sudden death in epilepsy: forensic and clinical issues*, CRC Press, Boca Raton, pp. 37-55.

Leestma, JE, Walczak, T, Hughes, JR, Kalelkar, MB & Teas, SS 1989, 'A prospective study on sudden unexpected death in epilepsy', *Ann Neurol*, vol. 26, no. 2, pp. 195-203.

Lehnertz, K, Mormann, F, Osterhage, H, Muller, A, Prusseit, J, Chernihovskyi, A, Staniek, M, Krug, D, Bialonski, S & Elger, CE 2007, 'State-of-the-art of seizure prediction', *J Clin Neurophysiol*, vol. 24, no. 2, pp. 147-53.

Lewis, S, Higgins, S & Goodwin, M 2008, 'Informing patients about sudden unexpected death in epilepsy: a survey of specialist nurses', *British Journal of Neuroscience Nursing*, vol. 4, no. 1, pp. 30-4.

Lhatoo, SD, Faulkner, HJ, Dembny, K, Trippick, K, Johnson, C & Bird, JM 2010, 'An electroclinical case-control study of sudden unexpected death in epilepsy', *Ann Neurol*, vol. 68, no. 6, pp. 787-96

Lim, EC, Lim, SH & Wilder-Smith, E 2000, 'Brain seizes, heart ceases: a case of ictal asystole', *J Neurol Neurosurg Psychiatry*, vol. 69, no. 4, pp. 557-9..

Lucas, SB, Cooper, H, Emmett, S, Hargraves, C & Mason, M 2006, *The conroner's autopsy: do we deserve better?*, National Confidential Enquiry into Patient Outcome and Death (NCEPOD), London.

MacCormick, JM, McAlister, H, Crawford, J, French, JK, Crozier, I, Shelling, AN, Eddy, CA, Rees, MI & Skinner, JR 2009, 'Misdiagnosis of long QT syndrome as epilepsy at first presentation', *Ann Emerg Med*, vol. 54, no. 1, pp. 26-32.

Mangena-Netshikweta, ML 2003, 'Perceptions about epilepsy in the Limpopo Province of the Republic of South Africa', *Curationis*, vol. 26, no. 4, pp. 51-6.

McCoy, D, Labonte, R, Walt, G, Sanders, D, Ram, R, Luppe, T, Germain, A & Dare, L 2011, 'The IHP+: a welcome initiative with an uncertain future', *Lancet*, vol. 377, no. 9780, pp. 1835-6.

McSharry, PE, Smith, LA & Tarassenko, L 2003, 'Comparison of predictability of epileptic seizures by a linear and a nonlinear method', *IEEE Trans Biomed Eng*, vol. 50, no. 5, pp. 628-33.

Meinardi, H, Scott, RA, Reis, R & Sander, JW 2001, 'The treatment gap in epilepsy: the current situation and ways forward', *Epilepsia*, vol. 42, no. 1, pp. 136-49.

Meyer, S, Shamdeen, MG, Gottschling, S, Strittmatter, M & Gortner, L 2011, 'Sudden unexpected death in epilepsy in children', *J Paediatr Child Health*, vol. 47, no. 6, pp. 326-31.

Mittan, R 1986, 'Fear of seizures', in S Whitman & B Hermann (eds), *Psychopathology in epilepsy: social dimensions*, Oxford University Press, New York, pp. 90-121.

Mohanraj, R, Norrie, J, Stephen, LJ, Kelly, K, Hitiris, N & Brodie, MJ 2006, 'Mortality in adults with newly diagnosed and chronic epilepsy: a retrospective comparative study', *Lancet Neurol*, vol. 5, no. 6, pp. 481-7.

Monte, CP, Arends, JB, Tan, IY, Aldenkamp, AP, Limburg, M & de Krom, MC 2007, 'Sudden unexpected death in epilepsy patients: Risk factors. A systematic review', *Seizure,* vol. 16, no. 1, pp. 1-7.

Morgan, MG, Fischhoff, B, Bostrom, A & Atman, C 2002, *Risk comunication: a mental models approach*, Cambridge University Press, Cambridge.

Mormann, F, Andrzejak, RG, Elger, CE & Lehnertz, K 2007, 'Seizure prediction: the long and winding road', *Brain*, vol. 130, Pt 2, pp. 314-33.

Mormann, F, Andrzejak, RG, Kreuz, T, Rieke, C, David, P, Elger, CE & Lehnertz, K 2003, 'Automated detection of a preseizure state based on a decrease in synchronization in intracranial electroencephalogram recordings from epilepsy patients', *Phys Rev E Stat Nonlin Soft Matter Phys*, vol. 67, no. 2 Pt 1, p. 021912.

Morton, B, Richardson, A & Duncan, S 2009, 'Sudden unexpected death in epilepsy: don't ask, don't tell?', *J Neurol Neurosurg Psychiatry*, vol. 77, pp. 199-202.

Mukherjee, S, Tripathi, M, Chandra, PS, Yadav, R, Choudhary, N, Sagar, R, Bhore, R, Pandey, RM & Deepak, KK 2009, 'Cardiovascular autonomic functions in well-controlled and intractable partial epilepsies', *Epilepsy Res*, vol. 85, no. 2-3, pp. 261-9.

Nashef, L 1997, 'Sudden unexpected death in epilepsy: terminology and definitions', *Epilepsia*, vol. 38, Suppl 11, pp. S6-8.

Nashef, L, Annegers, JF & Brown, SW 1997, 'Introduction and Overview', *Epilepsia*, vol. 38, Suppl 11, pp. S1-S2.

Nashef, L, Fish, DR, Garner, S, Sander, JW & Shorvon, SD 1995, 'Sudden death in epilepsy: a study of incidence in a young cohort with epilepsy and learning difficulty', *Epilepsia*, vol. 36, no. 12, pp. 1187-94.

Nashef, L & Ryvlin, P 2009, 'Sudden unexpected death in epilepsy (SUDEP): update and reflections', *Neurol Clin*, vol. 27, no. 4, pp. 1063-74.

Nashef, L, So, EL & Tomson, T 'Definition of sudden unexpected death in epilepsy (SUDEP): a clinical category rather than a syndrome (in preparation)'.

National Health Service National Clinical Health Outcomes Knowledge Base (NCHOD) 2009, Years of life lost due to mortality from epilepsy, viewed June 18 2011, <http://www.nchod.nhs.uk/NCHOD/compendium.nsf/17b8958892856d44802573a30020fcd9/a8edc5d0aa7577a6652573b200151bb4!OpenDocument>.

Ndiaye, M, Sene-Diouf, F, Diop, AG & Ndiaye, IP 2000, 'Epilepsy: first-ranked disorder in pediatric services of Senegal', *Bull Soc Pathol Exot*, vol. 93, no. 4, pp. 268-9.

Nei, M & Bagla, R 2007, 'Seizure-related injury and death', *Curr Neurol Neurosci Rep*, vol. 7, no. 4, pp. 335-41.

Nickels, K & Wirrell, E 2010, Epilepsy-related mortality is low in children: a 25 year polulation-based study in Rochester, MN (abstract), American Epilepsy Society (AES), viewed Feb 12 2010, <http://www.aesnet.org/go/publications/aes-abstracts/abstract-search/mode/display/st/mortality/sy/2010/sb/All/id/12940>.

Nilsson, L, Ahlbom, A, Farahmand, BY & Tomson, T 2003, 'Mortality in a population-based cohort of epilepsy surgery patients', *Epilepsia*, vol. 44, no. 4, pp. 575-81.

Nilsson, L, Farahmand, BY, Persson, PG, Thiblin, I & Tomson, T 1999, 'Risk factors for sudden unexpected death in epilepsy: a case-control study', *Lancet*, vol. 353, no. 9156, pp. 888-93.

Nolte, E & McKee, M 2004, *Does health care save lives? Avoidable mortality revisited*, The Nuffield Trust, London.

Persson, H, Kumlien, E, Ericson, M & Tomson, T 2005, 'Preoperative heart rate variability in relation to surgery outcome in refractory epilepsy', *Neurology*, vol. 65, no. 7, pp. 1021-5.

Persson, H, Kumlien, E, Ericson, M & Tomson, T 2007, 'Circadian variation in heart-rate variability in localization-related epilepsy', *Epilepsia*, vol. 48, no. 5, pp. 917-22.

Pijn, JP, Van Neerven, J, Noest, A & Lopes da Silva, FH 1991, 'Chaos or noise in EEG signals; dependence on state and brain site', *Electroencephalogr Clin Neurophysiol*, vol. 79, no. 5, pp. 371-81.

Pritchard, WS & Duke, DW 1995, 'Measuring "chaos" in the brain: a tutorial review of EEG dimension estimation', *Brain Cogn*, vol. 27, no. 3, pp. 353-97.

Puvanendran, K 1993, 'Epidemiology of epilepsy in Singapore', *Ann Acad Med Singapore*, vol. 22, Suppl 3, pp. 489-92.

Rajna, P, Clemens, B, Csibri, E, Dobos, E, Geregely, A, Gottschal, M, Gyorgy, I, Horvath, A, Horvath, F, Mezofi, L, Velkey, I, Veres, J & Wagner, E 1997, 'Hungarian multicentre epidemiologic study of the warning and initial symptoms (prodrome, aura) of epileptic seizures', *Seizure*, vol. 6, no. 5, pp. 361-8.

Raphael, B 1977, 'Preventative intervention with the recently bereaved', *Arch Gen Psychiatry*, vol. 34, no. 12, pp. 1450-4.

Redhead, K, Tasker, P, Suchak, K, Ahmed, M, Copsey, G, Roberts, P, Daws, J & Titmarsh, M 1996, 'Audit of the care of patients with epilepsy in general practice', *Br J Gen Pract*, vol. 46, no. 413, pp. 731-4.

Richerson, GB 2004, 'Serotonergic neurons as carbon dioxide sensors that maintain pH homeostasis', *Nat Rev Neurosci*, vol. 5, no. 6, pp. 449-61.

Richerson, GB & Buchanan, GF 2011, 'The serotonin axis: Shared mechanisms in seizures, depression, and SUDEP', *Epilepsia*, vol. 52, pp. 28-38.

Ridsdale, L, Charlton, J, Ashworth, M, Richardson, MP & Gulliford, MC 2011, 'Epilepsy mortality and risk factors for death in epilepsy: a population-based study', *Br J Gen Pract*, vol. 61, no. 586, pp. 271-8.

Rosenfeld, WE, Bramley, TJ & Meyer, KL 2004, 'Patient compliance with topiramate vs. other antiepileptic drugs: a claims database analysis', , vol. 45, Suppl 7, Abstract 2.141.

Rossetti, AO, Dworetzky, BA, Madsen, JR, Golub, O, Beckman, JA & Bromfield, EB 2005, 'Ictal asystole with convulsive syncope mimicking secondary generalisation: a depth electrode study', *J Neurol Neurosurg Psychiatry*, vol. 76, no. 6, pp. 885-7.

Royal College of Pathology (RCP) Working Party on the Autopsy 2005, *Guidelines on autopsy practice: scenario 6 - deaths associated with epilepsy*, The Royal College of Pathologists, London.

Rugg-Gunn, FJ, Simister, RJ, Squirrell, M, Holdright, DR & Duncan, JS 2004, 'Cardiac arrhythmias in focal epilepsy: a prospective long-term study', *Lancet*, vol. 364, no. 9452, pp. 2212-9.

Ryvlin, P & Kahane, P 2003, 'Does epilepsy surgery lower the mortality of drug-resistant epilepsy?', *Epilepsy Res*, vol. 56, no. 2-3, pp. 105-20.

Ryvlin, P, Tomson, T & Montavont, A 2009, '[Excess mortality and sudden unexpected death in epilepsy] [article in French]', *Presse Med*, vol. 38, no. 6, pp. 905-10.

Sakamoto, K, Saito, T, Orman, R, Koizumi, K, Lazar, J, Salciccioli, L & Stewart, M 2008, 'Autonomic consequences of kainic acid-induced limbic cortical seizures in rats: peripheral autonomic nerve activity, acute cardiovascular changes, and death', *Epilepsia*, vol. 49, no. 6, pp. 982-96.

Salanova, V, Markand, O & Worth, R 2002, 'Temporal lobe epilepsy surgery: outcome, complications, and late mortality rate in 215 patients', *Epilepsia*, vol. 43, no. 2, pp. 170-4.

Salanova, V, Markand, O & Worth, R 2005, 'Temporal lobe epilepsy: analysis of failures and the role of reoperation', *Acta Neurol Scand*, vol. 111, no. 2, pp. 126-33.

Schimpf, R, Borggrefe, M & Wolpert, C 2008, 'Clinical and molecular genetics of the short QT syndrome', *Curr Opin Cardiol*, vol. 23, no. 3, pp. 192-8.

Schouten, EG, Dekker, JM, Meppelink, P, Kok, FJ, Vandenbroucke, JP & Pool, J 1991, 'QT interval prolongation predicts cardiovascular mortality in an apparently healthy population', *Circulation*, vol. 84, no. 4, pp. 1516-23.

Schraeder, PL, Delin, K, McClelland, RL & So, EL 2006, 'Coroner and medical examiner documentation of sudden unexplained deaths in epilepsy', *Epilepsy Res*, vol. 68, no. 2, pp. 137-43.

Schraeder, PL, Delin, K, McClelland, RL & So, EL 2009, 'A nationwide survey of the extent of autopsy in sudden unexplained death in epilepsy', *Am J Forensic Med Pathol*, vol. 30, no. 2, pp. 123-6.

Schuele, SU, Bermeo, AC, Alexopoulos, AV, Locatelli, ER, Burgess, RC, Dinner, DS & Foldvary-Schaefer, N 2007, 'Video-electrographic and clinical features in patients with ictal asystole', *Neurology*, vol. 69, no. 5, pp. 434-41.

Schuele, SU, Widdess-Walsh, P, Bermeo, A & Luders, HO 2007, 'Sudden unexplained death in epilepsy: the role of the heart', *Cleve Clin J Med*, vol. 74, Supp 1, pp. S121-7.

Schuele, SU, Bermeo, AC, Locatelli, E, Burgess, RC & Luders, HO 2008, 'Ictal asystole: a benign condition?', *Epilepsia*, vol. 49, no. 1, pp. 168-71.

Schulze-Bonhage, A & Kuhn, A 2008, 'Unpredictability of seizures and the burden of epilepsy', in B Schelter, J Timmer & A Schulze-Bonhage (eds), *Seizure prediction in epilepsy*, WILEY-VCH Verlag GmbH & Co. KGaA, Weinheim.

Scorza, FA, Arida, RM, Terra, VC & Cavalheiro, EA 2010, 'What can be done to reduce the risk of SUDEP?', *Epilepsy Behav*, vol. 18, no. 3, pp. 137-8.

Scorza, FA, Colugnati, DB, Pansani, AP, Sonoda, EY, Arida, RM & Cavalheiro, EA 2008, 'Preventing tomorrow's sudden cardiac death in epilepsy today: what should physicians know about this?', *Clinics (Sao Paulo)*, vol. 63, no. 3, pp. 389-94.

Scottish Intercollegiate Guidelines Network 2003, *Diagnosis and Management of Epilepsy in Adults*, Scottish Intercollegiate Guidelines Network, Edinburgh.

Seyal, M & Bateman, LM 2009, 'Ictal apnea linked to contralateral spread of temporal lobe seizures: Intracranial EEG recordings in refractory temporal lobe epilepsy', *Epilepsia*, vol. 50, no. 12, pp. 2557-62.

Seyal, M, Bateman, LM, Albertson, TE, Lin, TC & Li, CS 2010, 'Respiratory changes with seizures in localization-related epilepsy: analysis of periictal hypercapnia and airflow patterns', *Epilepsia*, vol. 51, no. 8, pp. 1359-64.

Seyal, M, Pascual, F, Lee, CYM, Li, CS & Bateman, LM 2011, 'Seizure-related cardiac repolarization abnormalities are associated with the depth and duration of ictal hypoxemia', *Epilepsia*, In Press.

Shen, HY, Li, T & Boison, D 2010, 'A novel mouse model for sudden unexpected death in epilepsy (SUDEP): role of impaired adenosine clearance', *Epilepsia*, vol. 51, no. 3, pp. 465-8.

Shinnar, S, O'Dell, C & Berg, AT 2005, 'Mortality following a first unprovoked seizure in children: a prospective study', *Neurology*, vol. 64, no. 5, pp. 880-2.

Shorvon, S & Tomson, T 2011, 'Sudden unexpected death in epilepsy', *Lancet*, Jul 5 [Epub ahead of print].

SIGN see Scottish Intercollegiate Guidelines Network.

Sillanpää, M, Jalava, M, Kaleva, O & Shinnar, S 1998, 'Long-term prognosis of seizures with onset in childhood', *N Engl J Med*, vol. 338, no. 24, pp. 1715-22.

Sillanpää, M & Shinnar, S 2010, 'Long-term mortality in childhood-onset epilepsy', *N Engl J Med*, vol. 363, no. 26, pp. 2522-9.

Snow, RW, Williams, RE, Rogers, JE, Mung'ala, VO & Peshu, N 1994, 'The prevalence of epilepsy among a rural Kenyan population: its association with premature mortality', *Trop Geogr Med*, vol. 46, no. 3, pp. 175-9.

So, EL 2008, 'What is known about the mechanisms underlying SUDEP?', *Epilepsia*, vol. 49, Supp 9, pp. 93-8.

So, EL, Bainbridge, J, Buchhalter, JR, Donalty, J, Donner, EJ, Finucane, A, Graves, NM, Hirsch, LJ, Montouris, GD, Temkin, NR, Wiebe, S & Sierzant, TL 2009, 'Report of the American Epilepsy Society and the Epilepsy Foundation Joint Task Force on Sudden Unexplained Death in Epilepsy', *Epilepsia*, vol. 50, no. 4, pp. 917-22.

So, NK & Sperling, MR 2007, 'Ictal asystole and SUDEP', *Neurology*, vol. 69, no. 5, pp. 423-4.

Sperling, MR 2004, 'The consequences of uncontrolled epilepsy', *CNS Spectr*, vol. 9, no. 2, pp. 98-101, 6-9.

Sperling, MR, Feldman, H, Kinman, J, Liporace, JD & O'Connor, MJ 1999, 'Seizure control and mortality in epilepsy', *Ann Neurol*, vol. 46, no. 1, pp. 45-50.

Sperling, MR, Harris, A, Nei, M, Liporace, JD & O'Connor, MJ 2005, 'Mortality after epilepsy surgery', *Epilepsia*, vol. 46 Suppl 11, pp. 49-53.

Spratling, WP 1904, 'Prognosis', in Epilepsy and its treatment, W. B. Saunders, Philadelphia, p. 304.

Stavem, K & Guldvog, B 2005, 'Long-term survival after epilepsy surgery compared with matched epilepsy controls and the general population', *Epilepsy Res*, vol. 63, no. 1, pp. 67-75.

Stokes, T, Shaw, EJ, Juarez-Garcia, A, Camosso-Stefinovic, J & Baker, R 2004, *Clinical guidelines and evidence review for the epilepsies: diagnosis and management in adults and children in primary and secondary care*, Royal College of General Practitioners (RCGP).

Sundewall, J, Swanson, RC, Betigeri, A, Sanders, D, Collins, TE, Shakarishvili, G & Brugha, R 2011, 'Health-systems strengthening: current and future activities', *Lancet*, vol. 377, no. 9773, pp. 1222-3.

Surges, R, Taggart, P, Sander, JW & Walker, MC 2010, 'Too long or too short? New insights into abnormal cardiac repolarization in people with chronic epilepsy and its potential role in sudden unexpected death', *Epilepsia*, vol. 51, no. 5, pp. 738-44.

Surges, R, Thijs, RD, Tan, HL & Sander, JW 2009, 'Sudden unexpected death in epilepsy: risk factors and potential pathomechanisms', *Nat Rev Neurol*, vol. 5, no. 9, pp. 492-504.

Tan, CT 2007, 'Differences in epilepsy and seizures between Asia and the West', *Neurology Asia*, vol. 12, pp. 59-60.

Tao, JX, Qian, S, Baldwin, M, Chen, XJ, Rose, S, Ebersole, SH & Ebersole, JS 2010, 'SUDEP, suspected positional airway obstruction, and hypoventilation in postictal coma', *Epilepsia*, vol. 51, no. 11, pp. 2344-7.

Teh, H, Tan, HJ, Loo, C & Raymonf, AA 2007, 'Short QT in Malaysian population', *Medical Journal or Malaysia*, vol. 62, pp. 10428.

Tekle-Haimanot, R, Forsgren, L & Ekstedt, J 1997, 'Incidence of epilepsy in rural central Ethiopia', *Epilepsia*, vol. 38, no. 5, pp. 541-6.

Tellez-Zenteno, JF, Ronquillo, LH & Wiebe, S 2005, 'Sudden unexpected death in epilepsy: evidence-based analysis of incidence and risk factors', *Epilepsy Res*, vol. 65, no. 1-2, pp. 101-15.

Terra, VC, Arida, RM, Rabello, GM, Cavalheiro, EA & Scorza, FA 2011, 'The utility of omega-3 fatty acids in epilepsy: more than just a farmed tilapia!', *Arq Neuropsiquiatr,* vol. 69, no. 1, pp. 118-21.

Terra, VC, Scorza, FA, Sakamoto, AC, Pinto, KG, Fernandes, RM, Arida, RM, Cavalheiro, EA & Machado, HR 2009, 'Does sudden unexpected death in children with epilepsy occur more frequently in those with high seizure frequency?', *Arq Neuropsiquiatr*, vol. 67, no. 4, pp. 1001-2.

Tomson, T, Nashef, L & Ryvlin, P 2008, 'Sudden unexpected death in epilepsy: current knowledge and future directions', *Lancet Neurol*, vol. 7, no. 11, pp. 1021-31.

Toth, V, Hejjel, L, Fogarasi, A, Gyimesi, C, Orsi, G, Szucs, A, Kovacs, N, Komoly, S, Ebner, A & Janszky, J 2010, 'Periictal heart rate variability analysis suggests long-term postictal autonomic disturbance in epilepsy', *Eur J Neurol,* vol. 17, no. 6, pp. 780-7.

Tran, DS, Odermatt, P, Le, TO, Huc, P, Druet-Cabanac, M, Barennes, H, Strobel, M & Preux, PM 2006, 'Prevalence of epilepsy in a rural district of central Lao PDR', *Neuroepidemiology*, vol. 26, no. 4, pp. 199-206.

Tran, DS, Zen, J, Strobel, M, Odermatt, P, Preux, PM, Huc, P, Delneuville, L & Barennes, H 2008, 'The challenge of epilepsy control in deprived settings: low compliance and high fatality rates during a community-based phenobarbital program in rural Laos', *Epilepsia*, vol. 49, no. 3, pp. 539-40.

Trans-Tasman Response AGAinst Sudden Death in the young (TRAGADY) 2008, Post-mortem in sudden unexpected death in the young: guidelines on autopsy practice, viewed July 13 2011, <http://www.rcpa.edu.au/static/File/Asset%20library/public%20 documents/ExternalOrganisations/Protocol%20for%20TRAGADY.pdf>.

Tu, E, Bagnall, RD, Duflou, J & Semsarian, C 2011, 'Post-mortem review and genetic analysis of sudden unexpected death in epilepsy (SUDEP) cases', *Brain Pathol*, vol. March 2, no. 2, pp. 201-8.

Tupal, S & Faingold, CL 2006, 'Evidence supporting a role of serotonin in modulation of sudden death induced by seizures in DBA/2 mice', *Epilepsia*, vol. 47, no. 1, pp. 21-6.

UK Parliamentary Debates October 12 2010, House of Commons, columns 1-43, viewed July 10 2011, http://www.publications.parliament.uk/pa/cm201011/cmhansrd/ cm101012/halltext/101012h0001.htm <http://www.parliamentlive.tv/Main/Player. aspx?meetingId=6591&st=09:30:19.>.

Uteshev, VV, Tupal, S, Mhaskar, Y & Faingold, CL 2010, 'Abnormal serotonin receptor expression in DBA/2 mice associated with susceptibility to sudden death due to respiratory arrest', Epilepsy Res, vol. 88, no. 2-3, pp. 183-8.

Walczak, T 2003, 'Do antiepileptic drugs play a role in sudden unexpected death in epilepsy?', *Drug Saf*, vol. 26, no. 10, pp. 673-83.

Walczak, TS, Leppik, IE, D'Amelio, M, Rarick, J, So, E, Ahman, P, Ruggles, K, Cascino, GD, Annegers, JF & Hauser, WA 2001, 'Incidence and risk factors in sudden unexpected death in epilepsy: a prospective cohort study', *Neurology*, vol. 56, no. 4, pp. 519-25.

Wang, WZ & Li, SC 1993, 'An extended test for community control of epilepsy proposed by WHO', *Chinese Journal of Nervous and Mental Diseases*, vol. 19, no. 1, pp. 16-9.

Wang, XF, Xiao, Z, Yan, Y, Lu, Y, Ma, ZH & Li, JP 2004, 'Clinical and pathological features of SUDEP', *Ch Journal of Neurology*, vol. 37, no. 6, pp. 495-8.

Wannamaker, BB 2011, 'Medicolegal and clinical experiences ', in CM Lathers, PL Schraeder, MW Bungo & JE Leestma (eds), *Sudden unexpected death in epilepsy: forensic and clinical issues*, CRC Press, Boca Raton, pp. 347-59.

Weber, P, Bubl, R, Blauenstein, U, Tillmann, BU & Lutschg, J 2005, 'Sudden unexplained death in children with epilepsy: a cohort study with an eighteen-year follow-up', *Acta Paediatr*, vol. 94, no. 5, pp. 564-7.

Wiebe, S, Blume, WT, Girvin, JP & Eliasziw, M 2001, 'A randomized, controlled trial of surgery for temporal-lobe epilepsy', *N Engl J Med*, vol. 345, no. 5, pp. 311-8.

Williams, J, Lawthom, C, Dunstan, FD, Dawson, TP, Kerr, MP, Wilson, JF & Smith, PE 2006, 'Variability of antiepileptic medication taking behaviour in sudden unexplained death in epilepsy: hair analysis at autopsy', *J Neurol Neurosurg Psychiatry*, vol. 77, no. 4, pp. 481-4.

Winterhalder, M, Maiwald, T, Voss, HU, Aschenbrenner-Scheibe, R, Timmer, J & Schulze-Bonhage, A 2003, 'The seizure prediction characteristic: a general framework to assess and compare seizure prediction methods', *Epilepsy Behav*, vol. 4, no. 3, pp. 318-25.

Wright, MA, Orth, M, Patsalos, PN, Smith, SJ & Richardson, MP 2006, 'Cortical excitability predicts seizures in acutely drug-reduced temporal lobe epilepsy patients', *Neurology*, vol. 67, no. 9, pp. 1646-51.

Yates, DW, Ellison, G & McGuiness, S 1990, 'Care of the suddenly bereaved', *BMJ*, vol. 301, no. 6742, pp. 29-31.

Yildiz, GU, Dogan, EA, Dogan, U, Tokgoz, OS, Ozdemir, K, Genc, BO & Ilhan, N 2011, 'Analysis of 24-hour heart rate variations in patients with epilepsy receiving antiepileptic drugs', *Epilepsy Behav*, vol. 20, no. 2, pp. 349-54.

Zhao, M, Suh, M, Ma, H, Perry, C, Geneslaw, A & Schwartz, TH 2007, 'Focal increases in perfusion and decreases in hemoglobin oxygenation precede seizure onset in spontaneous human epilepsy', *Epilepsia*, vol. 48, no. 11, pp. 2059-67.

Zielinski, JJ 1974, 'Epilepsy and mortality rate and cause of death', *Epilepsia*, vol. 15, no. 2, pp. 191-201.

notes

notes

notes